THE
DETOX LIFE

YOUR FOUR-WEEK GUIDE TO BETTER FITNESS, FAT LOSS AND ENHANCED ENERGY

Jaye
Thank you for
being for giving
so freely. We need
you. Upwards + Onwards
in 2020 ♡ Meth

NOW IS THE TIME FOR A FRESH START,

A NEW BEGINNING,

A REVITALIZATION IF YOU WILL...

COPYRIGHT

The information contained in this book is based on the research and experience of the author as a health and wellness professional. This book should not be used as a substitute for advice from your personal healthcare professionals. It is strongly recommended that readers consult with their private healthcare providers prior to engaging in any self-care or health-related practices specific to this guide or others.

Copyright © 2019 by Metra Lundy

Photography by Selina Garcia and David Bracetty
Cover design by Anya Semenova
Content editing by Elizabeth Bauchner
Production editing by Mario Maric
Copyediting by Cheryl Salerno
Recipes and food lists by Metra Lundy and others:
thejamicanmother.com, blog.fatfreevegan.com, minimalistbaker.com, theveglife.com, simpleveganblog.com, caribbeanpot.com, wholefully.com, tastebetterfromscratch.com, mommyshomecooking.com, foodnetwork.com, cookieandkate.com, veggierose.com, rawtarian.com, thespruceeats.com, lovingitvegan.com, natalienorman.com, simple-vegnista.com, thevegan8.com, veggieinspire.com, thespruceeats.com, veggiesdontbite.com, livesimplynatural.com, thefullhelping.com, aspicyperspective.com, elanapantry.com, runningonrealfood.com, draxe.com, eatingbirdfood.com, tastykitchen.com, southbeachdiet.com, Heal Thyself Natural Living Cookbook, wellnessmama.com

For more information please contact:

Inspire Me Fit LLC
Attn: Metra Lundy
PO Box 4576
Highland Park, NJ 08904

First e-book edition 2019
ISBN: 978-0-578-60164-9
Published by Metra Lundy

www.thedetoxlifebook.com
www.metralundy.com

ACKNOWLEDGEMENTS

This book is a product of the many lessons that have shaped me. Thank you to everyone who has ever added value to my life. I am grateful. I especially dedicate this text to my daughters Aniyah and Kamiylah and their unborn children. Thank you for teaching me how to love and nurture in a way that only an offspring is able to. Thank you to my mother Elaine for always being an example of determination and perseverance. To my siblings Al'Sakeena, Al'Nesa, Al'Shanell, Hamidullah and extended family members thank you for your many years of love and support. Finally, to my teachers, coaches, clients and friends thank you for always being a source of motivation and inspiration.

CONTENTS

APPENDIX   185

RECIPES   221

INTRODUCTION

Hello, I'm Metra Lundy, your own personal fitness professional and coach. I welcome you to the pages of this book with open arms and a smiling face. My goal is to help you shed weight (both physical and emotional), revitalize and renew. I have over ten years of experience guiding hundreds of clients like you through an exciting four-week program to detoxify their lives and start fresh. After reading this book and joining me on your detox journey, you'll have all the tools you need to engage in a simple, customized cleanse, as well as a personal workout regimen designed to improve your overall health, fitness, fat loss and energy . I will give you access to tons of delicious, nutrient-dense recipes that you can use anytime, as well as seven-day meal plans for every phase of your detox.

"The Detox Life" is divided into four parts: Think It, Eat It, Feel It, and Live It. Each section includes an overview, workout regimen, healthy recipes, menus, case studies, and advice for making detoxification part of the structure of your daily life. What is awesome about this plan is that you don't need to read it in consecutive order. Feel free to jump around to the areas that speak to your most pressing needs, but it's best to plan carefully before starting any new program. A book is not a replacement for medical advice, so please remember to consult with your healthcare professional before making any diet, exercise or lifestyle changes.

"The Detox Life" is perfect for people of all ages, sizes, genders, cultures, nationalities and abilities. I began to apply the tools I'm about to share with you over thirty years ago, and I am confident that with a little patience, hard work and sweat I can help you create a healthier, transformed version of yourself. Do turn each page with an open mind and an open heart.

Detoxification is a process, a journey that should be embarked upon with every change in the seasons. As your coach, I'd like to remind you that success is only relative to the goal that you are trying to accomplish. And, there really isn't a "wrong" way to detox as long as you are respecting, listening to and responding to your body. Hitting peaks and valleys isn't uncommon on a fitness and fat loss journey. Most of us have experienced times where we are either very committed to or very neglectful of our self-care. As a fitness coach, I see it all the time: an emotionally significant event like a marital engagement comes up, and boom! It sparks the idea to lose weight, work out and eat healthy. When the big day arrives, we look and feel amazing. Goal accomplished, awesome! But three weeks after that date, we're back to our old ways, and suddenly working out and eating healthy isn't our top priority. Our weight goes up, our motivation goes down and we are back at square one. Seasonal detoxification is a reinforcement tool. It says that we can remain at the top of the "fit and healthy mountain" as long as we maintain the initial habits that helped us get there in the first place.

Thirty to ninety days is the approximate length of time to fully adopt a new habit and see results that make us feel good about what we are doing. But, life is full of challenges, and the probability of undoing our success is high. The goal of a seasonal detox is to streamline our behaviors so that we can continuously and systematically live the best version of our healthy selves. When we detox seasonally, we are able to get in front of the predictable negative shifts that encourage us to consume more calories in the winter and fall, especially from comfort foods, and take advantage of the energy boost that comes in spring and summer, when we tend to eat light, drink more water and spend more time at parks and beaches for physical activity. Seasonal detoxification also reminds us to control our habits and behaviors and potentially control life-threatening conditions such as high blood pressure, blood insulin levels and cholesterol.

The act of detoxifying the way that we think, what we eat, how we feel and how we live is a journey, not a destination. Success on this journey means that we're always working on ourselves. I like to call it the ultimate house cleaning. "You" are the house that is constantly being cleaned, organized, renovated, reworked and refreshed. Because detoxifications are deliberate, they also tend to be deeply transformational.

How do you know when to detox? Consider a detox if:

1. You feel that you deserve to be happy and making positive changes to your wellbeing is a necessary step.

2. You feel that engaging in a detoxification may help to improve or eliminate one or more struggles you wish to tackle or are battling with.

3. You are prepared to address and work to overcome specific obstacles that might get in the way of you completing a successful detoxification.

Your first week of detoxification aims to help you shift your mindset. For seven days, you'll concentrate on bringing the positive into your life through the books you read, the movies you watch, the songs you listen to, the company you keep and the foods you eat.

It's time to lighten your load. Erykah Badu sings "Bag lady, you gone hurt your back draggin' all them bags like that. I bet nobody ever told you, all you should hold on to, is you, is you, is you...."

Now, whether you're a woman or man, the act of carrying too much stuff physically, mentally, emotionally and spiritually robs you of your motivation and brings you down.

The Detox Life is a lifestyle manual designed to positively affect:

- what and how you think

- what and how you eat

- how you feel

- and how you live day to day

In our first chapter together, "Think It", I'll give you a call to action and a goal for the week. You'll spend seven days focused on shifting your mindset, which I always say is 90% of the transformation game. And, what you will find is true is that you will need and want to take more than one week to work on letting go of the many things that we carry around. A week is not very long, but we have to begin somewhere. I encourage you to fuse the action items that work well for you into your everyday life for as long as you find them useful. In "Think It" I'll provide you with tips on bringing out the best version of yourself by sharing the experiences of real people and their success stories. I will coach you to choose foods that detoxify your mind and body so that you can think more clearly. You will receive positive reinforcement by way of quotes and short stories, a step-by-step read-it-and-eat-it meal plan and an "improve the way you think" workout of the week.

Whew! That was a lot. But the amazing news is that you can make this book a lifetime reference. Each time you read it you can take what you need, and skip what you are not ready for or don't want. By the way, I believe **YOU ARE A ROCK STAR** because you are willing to start with yourself to create positive change.

YOUR DAILY DETOXIFICATION REGIMEN

CLEAR
Remove that which no longer serves you

CLEANSE
Purify your internal and external environments

TRAIN
Workout most days of the week for 30-60 minutes

EAT WELL
Consume healthy, fresh foods, mostly plants in accordance with your chosen food level (Appendix Page 190)

LIVE
Implement "Live Life Tool" to help you better manage you

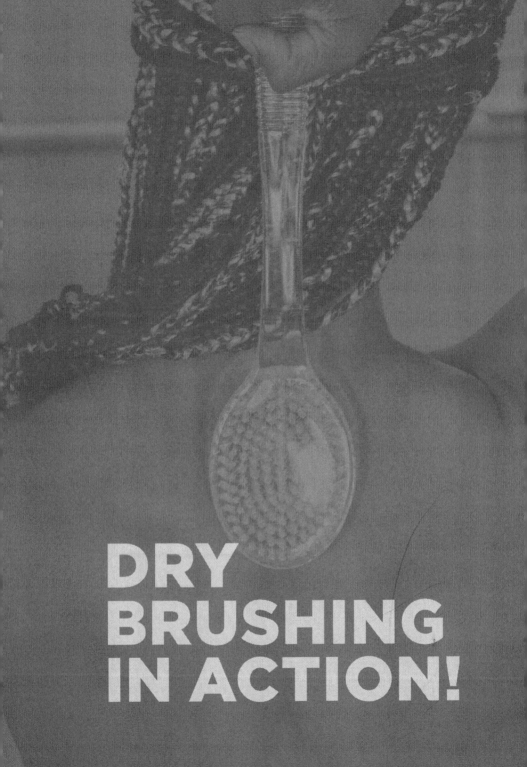

DRY BRUSHING IN ACTION!

What is dry body brushing?

Dry body brushing is the simple yet soothing action of brushing the body without water.

Why dry brush?

Some of the many benefits of dry brushing include improving the feel of the skin using exfoliation, stimulating blood circulation and reducing the appearance of cellulite all while maintaining your skin's moisture.

What is the symbolism of brushing?

Brushing the skin is great physical act but it can also be a symbolic act of renewal. Within the action we have the power to clean, clear or reawaken any surface of our bodies that we choose as well as remove any emotion, intention or mindset that no longer serves us.

Who should dry brush?

Anyone with healthy skin can dry brush. Areas of the skin that are irritated, bruised, broken, cut, inflamed or that are very sensitive should be avoided. Anyone with a life threatening illness should speak with their doctor before deciding to brush.

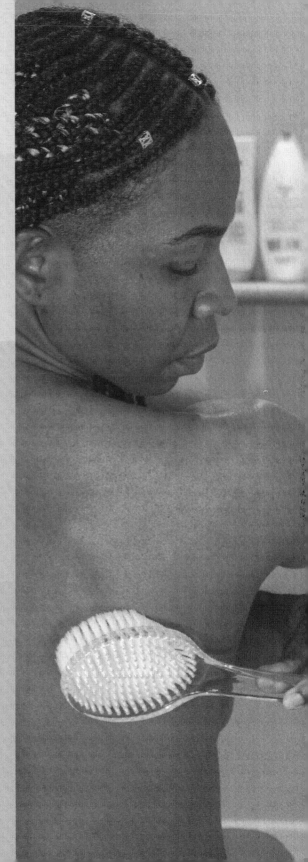

What type of brush should be used when dry brushing?

The desired bristle will vary from person to person but in general a medium stiff bristle brush works well for the body. A soft brush is better for the face or other areas where you would prefer softer stimulation. I use three different brushes—one for my body, one for my face and one for my back. Your back brush should have a long handle so that you can reach the areas of the back that are not easy to access.

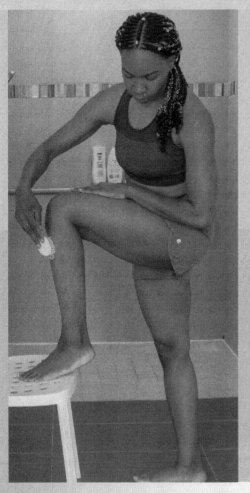

How should dry body brushing be done?

Brushing can be done from the bottom up or top down in a circular or upward direction. Be mindful that an exception to your brush direction can be made when trying to access hard to reach places such as your back. Do select the direction that creates the easiest execution.

How long should brushing take and when should it be done?

Brushing can take anywhere from ten to thirty minutes. It is most enjoyable when you have time to pay attention to how your body feels while brushing it. When possible, do shower when dry brushing is complete; it will rinse away the unwanted dead skin that was lifted during brushing.

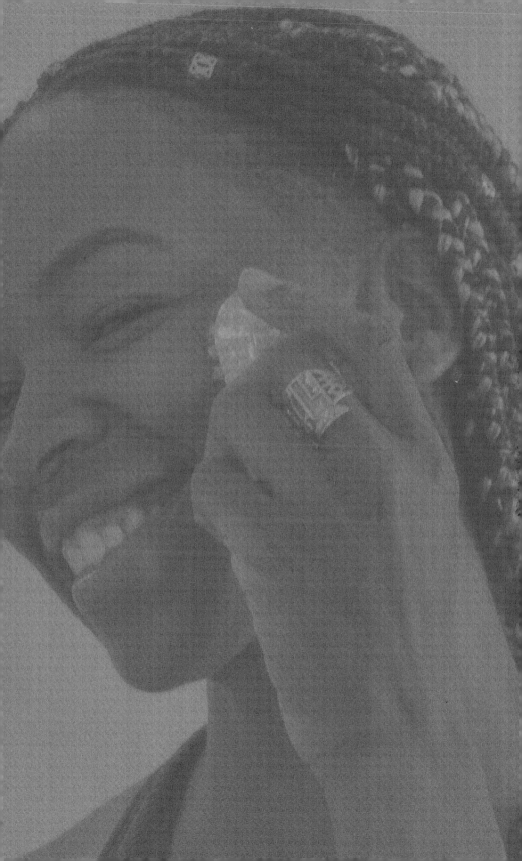

THINK IT!

THE POWER OF MENTAL DETOXIFICATION

She'd lost 100 Pounds

"Renewal requires opening yourself up to
new ways of thinking and feeling."

DEBORAH DAY

The day had been exceptionally busy. My office assistant had called out sick, I was alone and I'd finally gotten an opportunity to sit down to view the day's calendar. It felt like I'd done a full day of work, but it was only twelve o'clock. As I looked away from the clock and calendar on my phone, I saw an attractive woman approaching. With a little sass and a lot of curiosity she asked, "So what is this place?" I gave her my everyday gigantic coach smile and answered her question with a question. "Kinetics is a fitness and fat-loss facility; are you interested in either?" She was obviously overweight, but I didn't want to jump to any conclusions. With little hesitation, she told me that she had lost one hundred pounds over the last twelve months and was looking for help to lose her last one hundred. I responded, "Great, that is exactly what we do!" I asked whether she wanted one-on-one fitness training or to train with a small group. "I'm not sure," Alice said. "What you can tell me about either of them that might help me make up my mind?" So, I gave her a quick overview of how we help people get into the best shape of their lives. I spoke about personal training versus the group experience, and we both figured out right away that Alice would need to test the waters and experiment in order to decide which type of training would work best for her. I gave her my card, scheduled a follow-up session plus a one-week trial and sent her an email confirmation.

Alice was well-educated, confident and full of life. She had everything going for her except the one thing that had always been a problem in her life, her weight. Alice was one hundred and fifty pounds overweight. She had set a goal to lose one hundred of those pounds. When I mentioned the other fifty, she said, "Well, let's take off this hundred and then reassess. My goal is to also avoid looking sick, do you know what I mean?" I could tell that it was important to her that I know what she meant. I began her body analysis. "Part of my job, Alice, is to find out as much about you as possible. Tell me about your fitness background." With no sarcasm intended, Alice answered, "Ma'am, if I had a fitness background I wouldn't be talking to you now." We both smiled and got to her assessment exercises; step-ups, pushups, sit-ups, sit and reach, etc. I watched her move and listened carefully. "NO worries Alice, I will do my best to NOT ONLY help you lose the weight but get you feeling confident in your body as the weight comes off. By the time we are finished, nothing and no one is going to get in the way of you doing what you want, when you want, how you want." "Well," Alice said, "I like the way that sounds."

We finished by reviewing the details of her training plan. My suggestion was for her to do personal training. Alice was beautiful but obviously suffered from low self-confidence. From the time that she was a little girl she soothed her emotions with food. Growing up in a critical religious household had robbed her of the opportunity to learn self-love so instead she learned to love food instead. After all, food never spoke down to her; it was always available and it always made her feel good. Admitting all of this made Alice extremely vulnerable. She was embarrassed and ashamed of and didn't want the secrets of her suffering to be exposed. I could tell she needed privacy to work through her emotions, so personal training was the best option to jump-start her transformation.

Alice and I put in one full year of hard work. There was plenty of fussing and cussing on her end but together, we stayed committed to her goal. Alice had trained five days per week and kept a healthy mostly plant-based eating regimen for one full year. There was no going back. She was forever changed. Until today Alice has kept off the two hundred pounds that she originally lost. And, if you ever had the opportunity to meet her, she would tell you this (and I quote):

"It took me all of my life to believe that I could take this weight off. As soon as I understood that I needed to shift my way of thinking, my journey became much easier. I am a new person. I love the way I look and feel. I am forever changed."

Doesn't it feel amazing when we give ourselves permission to start over, and even better when that fresh start leads to a positive personal outcome? I have seen it time and time again with my clients and in myself. A special event is on the horizon, and we want to look and feel amazing for it. You know which events I'm referring to, right? An important wedding, a beach vacation, the birth of a child, or any other monumental occasion. Without a second thought, we start our healthy living journey over. We hone in and focus on how we want to BE for that special day. We get focused and take action, suddenly clean eating and workouts are less of a strain, and if we are serious we achieve our goals.

When we allow it to, detoxification helps us to slow down, get focused and start again.

So, what I would like for you to do now is to slow down and get focused:

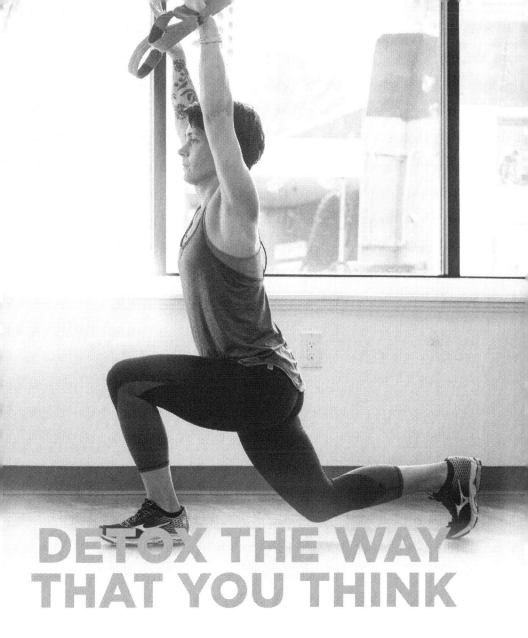

DETOX THE WAY THAT YOU THINK

YOUR COACH'S ADVICE:

Give everything you strive for your best effort. Stop complaining, and find a reason, big or small, to be excited about your life. Every day will feel monumentally more enjoyable.

LIVE LIFE TOOL

I encourage you to journal regularly; please keep your favorite notebook or stationary handy.

Most of us make decisions based on how we feel. To help manage your emotions write out your thoughts and feelings regularly. The hope is that writing it out will help you process life's challenges with more ease; you will work to accept what you cannot control and move forward. – Please pull out your journal now.

What do you want to accomplish overall during your detox?
What do you want to accomplish by the close of:
- Week one:
- Week two:
- Week three:
- Week four:

I want you to take control over creating a better you. I want you to know that you have the power and ability to slow down, focus, and press reset any time. As a matter of fact, I encourage you to STOP waiting for a special event and START working on improving around the clock. On the other side of that work is the opportunity for a happier, healthier, more fulfilling way of being in this world.

1. Daily, ask, "How am I feeling about myself?"
2. Weekly, establish what you aspire to improve
3. Quarterly, press reset on anything that is not working

Here is what is awesome. The glass is half full, not half empty, and the next seven days are in place to bring remarkable moments of fresh perspective and a healthier you.

Plan of action required

H e was seventy-five and recently married before he even considered exercising regularly. A life in construction work had kept him active but the injuries he'd incurred were now ailing concerns. His new wife was in her forties, active, energetic and driven; and he knew that she expected him to be the same way. After all, that is how he presented himself five years ago when they met. But it was obvious, he was slowing down and they both knew it.

"The doctor said that the arthritis will be less painful if you continue to move". Joe's wife gave a loving hug to her husband's arm. "Honey, you want me to start a workout regimen at my age. I have no clue about what to do; I don't need any injuries at my age". "My love", she responded. "I have a plan for you; we will prevent the likelihood that you will injure yourself by having you work with a trainer three times per week". He let out a "wow" of relief. "That's wonderful dear. Thank you for knowing that about me". She replied. "You are very welcome. However, I can't take all the credit. It was actually Judith, our therapist who made the recommendation. She casually mentioned it in our last session. The other thing that I did per her recommendation was to buy into one of the fresh meals on wheels companies. Starting tomorrow they will deliver healthy plant-based dinners and lunches for us to prepare at home since finding time to go to the grocery store has been a challenge for the both of us". "That's perfect, love. Making changes in this way seems much more sustainable", "I agree".

My gut feeling is that as long as we continue to support each other and seek the guidance of our experts, coaches, trainers, therapists and community of support, there is nothing that we can't handle at any age or condition.

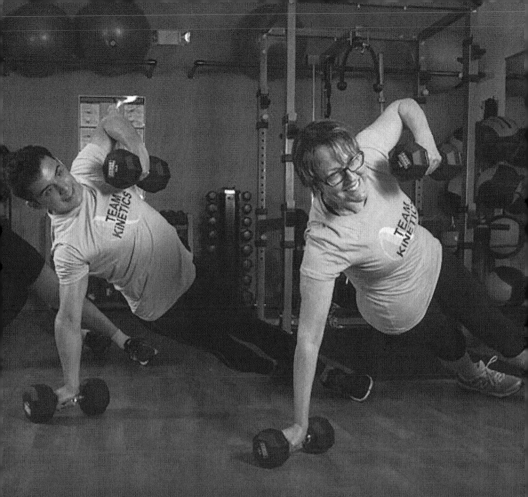

DETOX THE WAY
THAT YOU THINK

YOUR COACH'S ADVICE:

Be persistent in your quest for personal
improvement. Search for and implement
lifestyle strategies that yield a domino
effect of positive changes and outcomes.

ABOUT YOUR COACH

I have come to accept two very important, sometimes difficult realities in life. The only thing that's certain in this world is change; and the only person that I can control is me. I live The Detox Life because it teaches me how to adjust as the seasons, people and circumstances of my life change. It places the responsibility for how I think, what I eat, how I feel and how I live into my own hands. It places my personal power into my hands and allows me to live by my gratitude mantra:

- Today and every day I am grateful for a positive mindset and clarity of thought

- Today and every day I am grateful for foods that energize and give me life

- Today and every day I choose to feel good

- Today and every day I am living my best life

YOUR MANTRA

I am a gifted human being with a divine purpose in this world. In order to be and give my best, I must take care of myself. Today and everyday I choose the healthiest version of me.

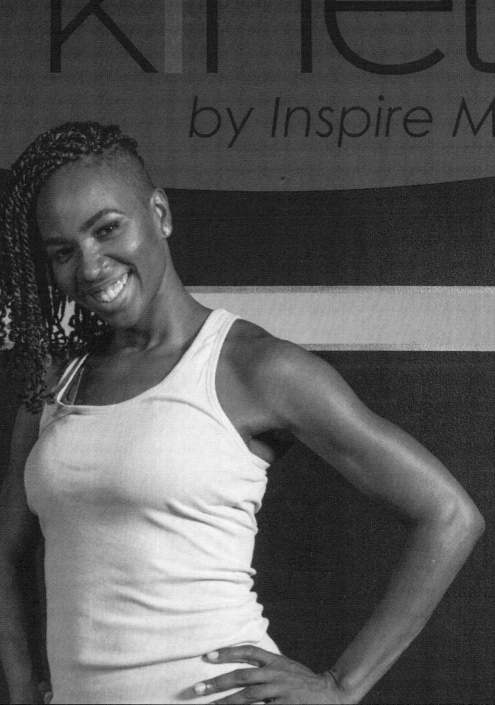

Who's that Guy in the Picture?

"Whatever you can do, or dream you can, begin it.
Boldness has genius, power and magic in it".

JOHANN WOLFGANG VON GOETHE

My flight to Las Vegas was a smooth one. I had gotten everything prepared for our 6-Week Body Transformation Challenge prior to leaving. We would be ready for our launch in two short days. I had a great feeling about this group. They were both anxious and excited to get started. Excitement is a must-have when it comes to any and all challenges! Lisa, one of our evening team leaders, called me as I was getting off the plane. Her voice was unusually high-pitched. "I just spoke with a guy who is really excited about the 6-week body transformation challenge. He had a lot of questions. I answered them for him, but he still wasn't sure if the program would be right for him. I know the challenge has closed, but I think that he would benefit greatly. He sounds so excited and willing. Can you call him?" "If you think that we can help him, please text me his number," I said, "and I'll give him a call now."

Tony-Tone answered on the second ring. His voice was strong and steady. "Yeah, I was looking at your place and I thought I might get some more information about what you do," he said, so I gave him our overview.

"We're a fitness and fat loss facility. What makes us unique is that we have four main areas of focus and they are MOTIVATION, ACCOUNTABILITY, HABIT and SAFETY." Tony-Tone listened but didn't seem moved, so I went on. "We guarantee results," I said. Tony-Tone's voice perked up. "How do you guarantee results?"

"Well, we give you a road map for fitness and fat-loss success. Then we implement check-in points to make sure that you stay on track with your goals; we are with you the entire time. Finally we are there to celebrate with you when your goals have been reached. And, if things get off track, we work with you to correct whatever is not working and get you moving full speed ahead towards your goals again. Tony-Tone," I said. "Are you ready to make a change for the better?"

From deep in his soul Tony-Tone roared, "YES!"

"Tony," I said, "Are you ready to make the changes that you've always wanted for your body come to life?" Tony-Tone roared, "YES!"

"But T," I said, "Are you ready to make this year the year that has you looking differently, behaving differently and living differently?" Tony-Tone used a football stadium roar again and said, "YES, let's do this!" I had a gigantic smile on my face, "Tony-Tone, dude, it's already done; we are only chugging through the motions." We hung up the phone but spoke once more that night. I could tell that he had given the initial call to me a lot of thought. He was ready.

Tony-Tone joined the 6-week body transformation challenge, and as I had guessed, he was hard core. Inspired by his own excitement and abilities, he went above and beyond the program requirements, training most days of the week, eating the food that was recommended and being content with the steady success that came along with that discipline. Tony dropped forty-two pounds, chiseled his arms and six-packed his abs. He came to us wanting to drop a few pounds and get healthy. What he got superceded what he thought he needed. It was a beautiful sight to see.

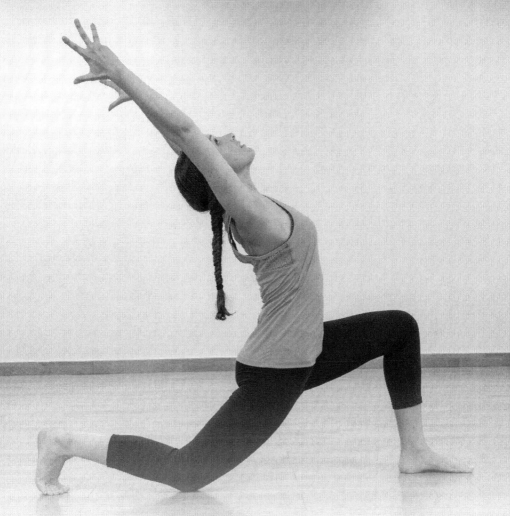

DETOX THE WAY THAT YOU THINK

YOUR COACH'S ADVICE:

What you think, speak and carry-out you become. Change your thoughts, words and actions then watch the possibility for new ways of experiencing the world surface.

LIVE LIFE TOOL

Music has the power to lift any mood. Allow this playlist to motivate you into healthy action or tap into another playlist that lightens your heads space and makes your energy soar.

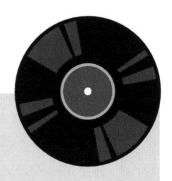

THINK IT PLAYLIST

- **Firework** by Katy Perry
- **I Wanna Rock** by Twisted Sister
- **Keep On Movin** by Soul II Soul
- **Shake It Off** by Taylor Swift
- **Push It Up** by DJ Drez Aficionados Instrumentals
- **It's My Life** by Bon Jovi
- **Something Just Like This** by The Chainsmokers & Coldplay
- **Meant To Be** by Bebe Rexha ft. Florida Georgia Line
- **Lose Yourself** by Eminem
- **Hit Me With Your Best Shot** by Pat Benatar

FITNESS TRAINING TIPS

I am beyond excited to be your Fitness Trainer for the first week of your detox. Remember that this is your journey not a race so DO pace yourself appropriately and modify your regimen when you feel that it is needed. In general I'd like for you to plan to be as active as possible, fitting in cardiovascular, strength, mobility and flexibility training every week.

FOR YOUR CARDIOVASCULAR TRAINING KEEP IN MIND THAT:

1. You have options! Enjoy walking, jogging, swimming, hiking and more

2. Your objective is to raise the heart rate to a level that feels challenging but not overwhelming

3. A great cardiovascular training minimum is most days of the week (five to six days) for 30 minutes

4. You'll start to feel the benefits from your cardiovascular training within a couple of weeks after you get started

FOR YOUR STRENGTH TRAINING KEEP IN MIND THAT:

1. You'll use your own body weight to build strength

2. You'll take a four-part approach to your workout, focusing on leg, push, hinge and pull exercises

3. A great strength training minimum is three days per week

4. You'll usually see and feel the benefits from strength work within four weeks of start of your training

FOR YOUR MOBILITY TRAINING
KEEP IN MIND THAT:

1. You'll focus on movements that encourage ease and a full range of motion at your joints

2. These movements are great when done at the beginning any workout

3. A great mobility training goal is most days of the week (five to seven days)

4. Benefits from mobility training are immediate

FOR YOUR FLEXIBILITY TRAINING
KEEP IN MIND THAT:

1. You'll focus on stretches that reduce stiffness and create long, healthy muscles

2. Stretches are great at the end of any workout

3. A great flexibility training goal is most days of the week (five to seven days)

4. Benefits from flexibility training are immediate

THINK IT!

Week One

LET'S GET YOU WARMED UP!

- Hit this workout at least **four days this week**. Our goal is to build your mental and physical strength!

- Do each movement for 30 – 60 seconds and repeat it two to three times before beginning your strength work.

- Make your movements as big as possible and go at a slow to medium pace.

SHOULDER ROLLS TO FULL ARM CIRCLES

- Roll your shoulders backwards five times, then forwards five times

- Fully extend your arms and create large arm circles, forwards five times each and then backwards five times

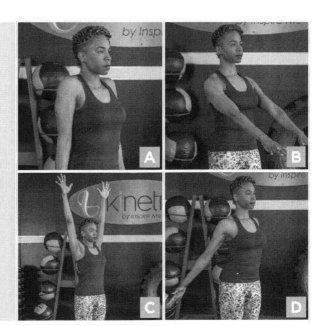

TORSO ROTATION

- Bring your arms to chest height

- Rotate your torso as far right and then as far left as you can

- Do your best to keep your hips facing forward

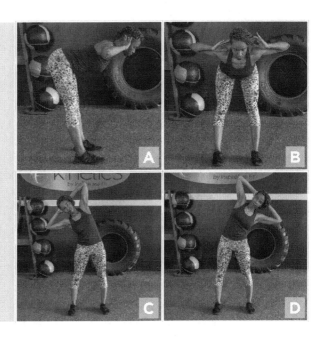

LATERAL LEG SWEEP

- Hold onto a sturdy surface

- Sweep one leg from the midline of your body out to the side of your body, and then repeat with the other leg

- Maintain a tall posture and engaged abs the entire time

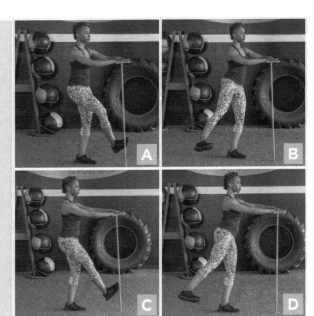

FORWARD LEG SWEEP

- Hold onto a sturdy surface

- Sweep one leg from the midline of your body forwards and backwards as high as you can, then repeat with the other leg

- Stand tall and engage your abs to avoid arching your back

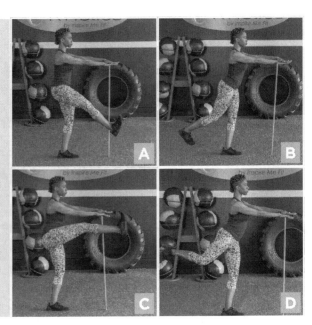

JUMPING JACKS

- Make this high or low impact

- Move with your arms fully extended

- Bring your legs together fully so that your ankles or inner thighs touch

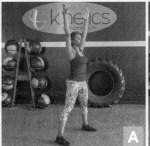
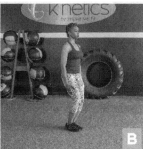
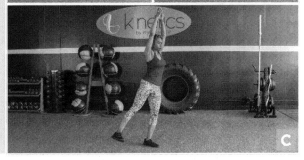

AWESOME JOB!

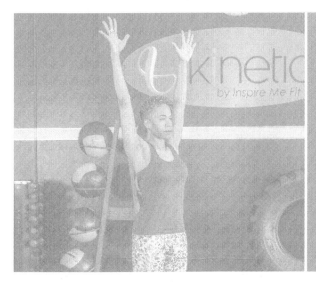

TIP OF THE DAY

Do each movement for 30 – 60 seconds and repeat it two to three times before beginning your strength work.

Make your movements as big as possible and go at a slow to medium pace.

STRENGTH WORKOUT

COMPLETE EXERCISES AS FOLLOWS:

- 30 seconds of work for beginners with a maximum of 60 seconds of rest between exercises

- 60 seconds of work for intermediate to advanced exercisers with no more than 30 seconds of rest between exercises

- 60 seconds of work for advanced exercisers with no rest between exercises

- Go in this order: legs, push, hinge and pull exercises. Complete two to four sets

- Complete one to two sets of cool-down exercises once your strength work is done

LEG EXERCISES

WALL SIT

- Put your upper back against the wall

- Plant your middle and lower back until you are in a seated position

- Hold steady

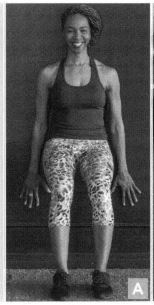
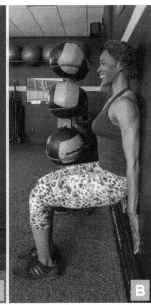

WARRIOR 3 REAR LEG LIFT

- Focus on balance

- Make sure your leg is fully extended

- Maintain a flat back

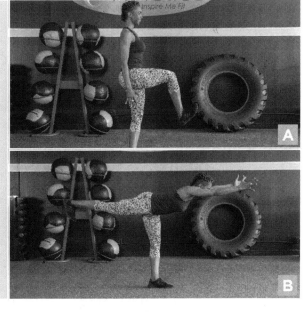

IN AND OUT SQUAT STEP

- Turn your toes out to one o'clock and eleven o'clock.

- Make sure that your knees and ankles align with your feet

- Sit back in your hips so that your knees don't pass over your toes

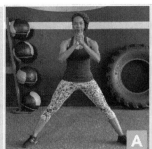
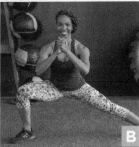
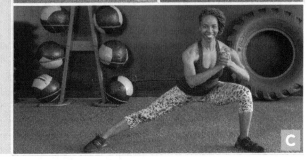

PUSH EXERCISES

PLANK WALKOUT TO PUSH-UP

- Begin in a standing position with the feet just beyond hip width apart.

- Transition into a squat, bring the hands up and place the elbows to the insides of the knees

- Walk out to a plank position

- Hit one to five push-ups per walkout

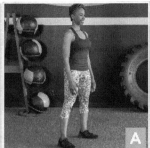
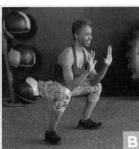
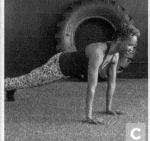
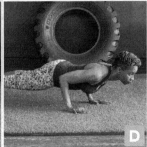

TRICEP DIPS

- Take a seat on any sturdy surface and keep your feet flush to the floor

- Align your hands on the surface so that they are shoulder-width

- Push your elbows behind you, aiming for a 90 degree angle

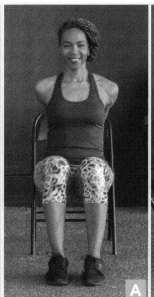
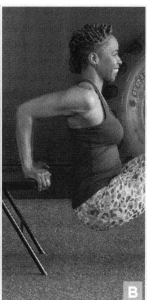

WALL PUSH OFF

- Assume a plank position on the wall

- Bend your elbows to push off

- Add a little fun by giving yourself a single, double or triple clap in between each push off

- Add more of a challenge by pushing off from a lower surface

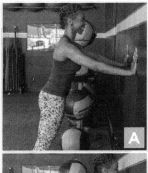
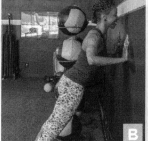
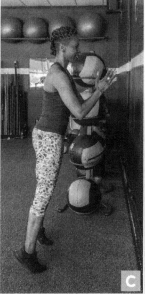

HINGE EXERCISES

SUPINE VERTICAL SCISSOR KICKS

- Plaster your low back to the floor

- Put a slight bend in your knees if you're unable to keep your legs up easily

- Exaggerate the distance between your legs

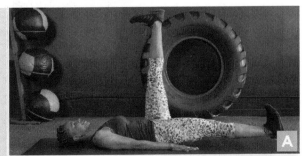
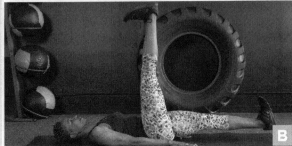

SUPINE BICYCLES

- When lifting your head, pull your shoulders forward and glue your low back to the floor

- Your head should feel heavy in your hands

- If your neck starts to bother you, push your tongue to the roof of your mouth to work the front neck muscles. Rest when needed

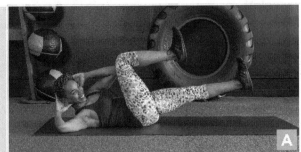
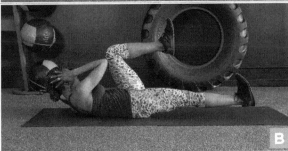

SUPINE CHAIR CRUNCH

- Plant your low back firmly

- Reach toward the ceiling, alternating your arms

- Feel the upper and middle abdominal muscles respond when the shoulders are lifted

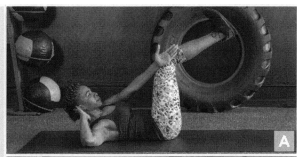

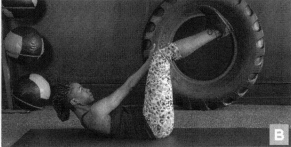

PULL EXERCISES

PRONE SUPER HERO

- Keep your feet planted

- Align your chin so that it's parallel to the floor

- Move your torso as you lift and lower your arms

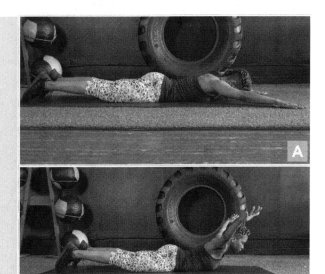

KNEELING LAT PULL-DOWN NO WALL SUPPORT

- This can be done with or without wall support

- For the straightest spinal alignment, support your upper, middle and low back flat against the wall

- Allow your head to float freely while you keep your arms flush to the wall

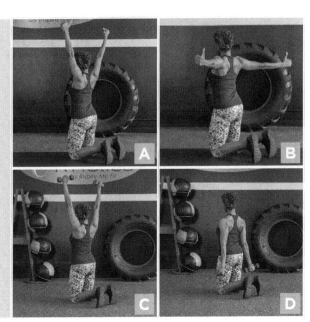

STANDING BENT OVER ROW

- Stand tall to begin. Push hips back and behind you. Roll the shoulders back and maintain a flat back

- Be sure to move your arms with maximum extension and retraction

- Engage your abs to help support your low back

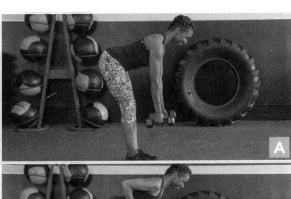
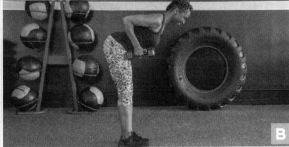

COOL-DOWN STRETCHES

YOGA CAT & COW

- Begin stretch with a neutral spine

- Round your back fully, looking towards your navel

- Drop your belly towards the floor while lifting your chest

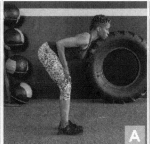
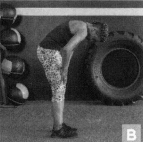
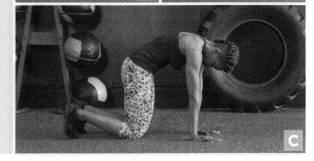

STANDING FORWARD BEND

- Stand tall, bringing your arms overhead

- As you bend, stretch your arms and chest as far forward as you can

- Once you are fully bent, allow your arms to relax and hang

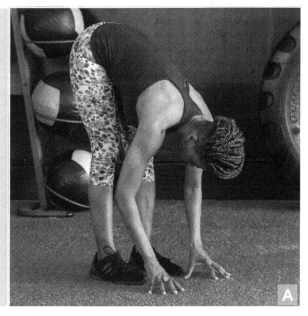

STANDING SIDE BEND

- Stand tall with both your legs and arms wide

- Bring alternating arms overhead as you stretch your side body

- Do your best to keep your hips and chest facing forward

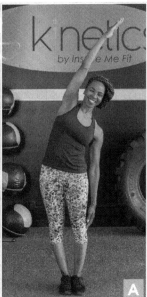

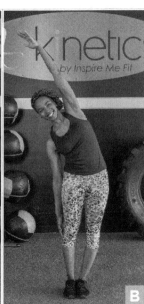

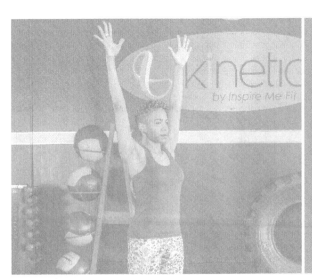

TIP OF THE DAY

Be aware: When exercising you will likely feel as if you're on the edge of discomfort but you should **NOT** be in pain.

If you're unsure of the difference between the two, **DO** reach out and I'll coach you through your next steps.

7 DAY READ IT AND EAT IT SAMPLE MENU FOR DETOXIFICATION

WEEK ONE:
YOUR ACTION ITEMS!

- Eat fresh, mostly plant-based foods in small portions preferably prepared in your own home

- Drink half your body weight in ounces of water (example if you're 140 lbs. drink 70 ounces of water)

- Monitor your sodium intake; consume no more than 2,000 milligrams daily

- Wean yourself away from sugar; consume no more than 24 grams of refined sugar per day and eat no more than 1-2 pieces of fresh fruit or one cup of fresh fruit juice daily.

- Read the labels on all packaged foods

- Eat foods with the fewest number of ingredients; aim for five ingredients or less

- Use this menu exactly as it is, choose leftovers instead of preparing a new meal or adjust food combinations.

- Your boost in energy as well as maintenance of a healthy weight will be achieved when you:
  » You eat consciously; knowing that everything that tastes good isn't good for you to eat
  » You eat real, whole foods that leave you feeling good
  » You eat lighter and a bit less than what you would normally eat

When your personal goals include losing weight or toning up, counting food calories helps tremendously. I am an advocate of counting calories because:

- You will be more aware of mindless eating

- Logging/tracking can be done by anyone, anytime and anywhere

- There are convenient websites and apps to help you calculate and monitor your caloric intake such as My Fitness Pal, Lose It or Fitbit

- An emphasis on tracking will lead to greater personal accountability

- Calorie counting does not require expensive tests or tools

- Calorie information is present on most nutrition packaging

A calorie is a unit of energy defined by the amount of heat required to raise 1 gram of water 1 degrees Celsius. In The Detox Life, when I talk about calories, I am referring to the energy that you will need to sustain your body while helping you maintain and/or lose weight. If weight loss is your goal, plan to use up more calories (energy) than you consume. A great goal would be for you to burn 250-500 calories daily via exercise routine.

DAY 1

Pre-Breakfast: 8 ounce glass of lemon or lime water, either warm or at room temperature

Breakfast: cream of quinoa, a serving of raw nuts and your choice of decaf coffee or tea

Lunch: easy vegan or fish tacos with your choice of a side salad

Dinner: lentil stew with your choice of a side salad

Snack options: sliced raw vegetables (avoid sweet vegetables like carrots or beets this week) and/or one serving of any non-sweet snack found in the snack recipes section. To achieve the best fat loss results, limit snack foods to 200 calories or less. Do your best to consume 64-80 ounces of water today while keeping your sodium intake to 2,000 mg total or less.

DAY 2

Pre-breakfast: 8 ounce glass of lemon or lime water, either warm or room temperature

Breakfast: omelet of your choice, sliced avocado and your choice of decaf coffee or tea

Lunch: zoodles with meatless meatballs, marinara sauce and your choice of side salad

Dinner: Grandma Flo's vegetable soup with a serving of almond crackers

Snack options: sliced raw vegetables (avoid sweet vegetables like carrots or beets this week) and/or one serving of any non-sweet snack found in the snack recipes section. To achieve the best fat loss results, limit snack foods to 200 calories or less. Do your best to consume 64-80 ounces of water today while keeping your sodium intake to 2,000mg total or less.

DAY 3

Pre-breakfast: 8 ounce glass of lemon or lime water, either warm or room temperature

Breakfast: protein shake of your choice, and your choice of either decaf coffee or tea

Lunch: vegetarian chili with your choice of side salad

Dinner: Asian vegetable stir fry with your choice of side salad

Snack options: sliced raw vegetables (avoid sweet vegetables like carrots or beets this week) and/or one serving of any non-sweet snack found in the snack recipes section. To achieve the best fat loss results, limit snack foods to 200 calories or less. Do your best to consume 64-80 ounces of water today while keeping your sodium intake to 2,000mg total or less.

DAY 4

Pre-breakfast: 8 ounce glass of lemon or lime water, either warm or room temperature

Breakfast: half cup cooked wake'um up oats and your choice of either decaf coffee or tea

Lunch: vegetarian eggplant parmesan with your choice of side salad

Dinner: steak of choice with your choice of a side salad

Snack options: sliced raw vegetables (avoid sweet vegetables like carrots or beets this week) and/or one serving of any non-sweet snack found in the snack recipes section. To achieve the best fat loss results, limit snack foods to 200 calories or less. Do your best to consume 64-80 ounces of water today while keeping your sodium intake to 2,000mg total or less.

DAY 5

Pre-Breakfast: 8 ounce glass of lemon or lime water either warm or room temperature

Breakfast: scrambled tofu or your choice omelet, sliced tomato and your choice of either decaf coffee or tea

Lunch: seasoned salmon, tofu or carrot tuna with your choice of a side salad

Dinner: open face lentil burger with your choice of a side salad

Snack options: sliced raw vegetables (avoid sweet vegetables like carrots or beets this week) and/or one serving of any non-sweet snack found in the snack recipes section. To achieve the best fat loss results, limit snack foods to 200 calories or less. Do your best to consume 64-80 ounces of water today while keeping your sodium intake to 2,000mg total or less.

DAY 6

Pre-breakfast: 8 ounce glass of lemon or lime water, either warm or room temperature

Breakfast: protein shake of choice and your choice of either decaf coffee or tea

Lunch: mashed cauliflower and meatless meatloaf with your choice of side salad

Dinner: curried vegetables with your choice of side salad

Snack options: sliced raw vegetables (avoid sweet vegetables like carrots or beets this week) and/or one serving of any non-sweet snack found in the snack recipes section. To achieve the best fat loss results, limit snack foods to 200 calories or less. Do your best to consume 64-80 ounces of water today while keeping your sodium intake to 2,000mg total or less.

DAY 7

Pre-breakfast: 8 ounce glass of lemon or lime water, either warm or room temperature

Breakfast: cream of quinoa, raw nuts and your choice of either coffee or tea

Lunch: healthy burrito and mixed greens

Dinner: steak with your choice of side salad

Snack options: sliced raw vegetables (avoid sweet vegetables like carrots or beets this week) and/or one serving of any non-sweet snack found in the snack recipes section. To achieve the best fat loss results, limit snack foods to 200 calories or less. Do your best to consume 64-80 ounces of water today while keeping your sodium intake to 2,000 mg total or less.

Congratulations! You did it, you made it through your first detoxification week. If you worked hard, thank you; I'm proud of you! If you chose not to work hard, know that this is a choice and you can do it. Don't let complacency keep you from crafting the best version of you. Great things are on the way; keep working! Your positive results will make all of this hard work worth it.

LIVE LIFE TOOL

Water is a powerful clear and cleanse element. Consider using water literally and symbolically to refresh and renew. As often as possible, take a soothing bath with the intention of removing that which no longer serves your mind, body and spirit. (Detox bath recipes Appendix page 188)

SECTION 2

EAT IT!

DETOXING WHAT YOU CONSUME

It's my wedding

"I often see how important it is to first believe that you can change your eating habits before you can make changes. If you want to eat mindfully, this is your first step. Tell yourself, 'It is not easy, but possible'"

DR. SUSAN ALBERS

"Listen, Metra," Amelia-Lynn spoke with a wholesome Latina accent. She had made up her mind. "I'm getting married in less than four months. Between my wedding and four of my best friend's weddings, I do not think that I will have time to get into shape." She gently hugged my shoulder with her left hand. "I need to look amazing for these weddings, especially mine! It is on the beach, you know!" Amelia poured out her background story. "My boyfriend and I run regularly, two to three times a week for thirty minutes. And, can you believe that over the last thirty days, he's dropped twelve pounds and I've only lost three? What is that about? Is there something wrong with me?"

"That is totally normal," I replied. "Men typically lose much faster than women." "I think that my body wants to hold on to all of this fat," she said, and grabbed her thighs. I opened my mouth to say something, but she continued passionately, "I need my stomach to be flat!" She pulled up her shirt and grabbed a roll of flesh at her waist. "This muffin top has got to go. My dress is sleeveless so I can't have jiggle underneath my arms. And this chin, there is a double one here."

I stopped her. "I have a few important questions for you in order to determine if your goal to be thinner, more toned and more beautiful for your wedding is possible. Is that okay?" "Of course," she responded. "One a scale of one to ten, can you rate yourself on the following questions with ten being a passionate yes and one being a definite no?" "Okay," she said.

"Would you say that you are a determined person?" "Yes, ten." "Okay; perfect!"

"When given specific instructions do you believe that you are capable of accomplishing any goal that you set for yourself?" "Will the instructions lead me to success?" "Yes!" "Well then, yes, and ten."

"Great, I have one final question. I am one-hundred percent certain that I can help you move the scale, get rid of your muffin top, tone up your arms and make you look and feel beautiful for your wedding. Will you allow me to coach you to success even knowing that there will be hard work and sweat involved?" Excitedly, she said, "Yes, and ten, that's why I'm here!" We both smiled and began working on her training plan.

Amelia-Lynn had thought about exactly what she wanted for herself. She'd claimed it, and sought out the help that she needed to make it happen. In three short months, Amelia-Lynn had dropped fifteen pounds. She had no more muffin top, and her arms were sexy and toned. She was ready for her wedding. Great intentions, a plan that worked and consistency led to her success. Amelia-Lynn was able to reach her goal to be fit, trim and feel beautiful for her wedding because she'd decided that she was unstoppable. She'd decided that she wanted to love the way she looked in her wedding pictures. Today, Amelia-Lynn has been married for a few years now. I asked her what specific actions she thought had led her to fat loss success. Her response was:

"It wasn't hard, but it also wasn't easy. It took me thinking differently about how I honor, respect and care for my body. My changes felt slow but steady; I had to come to terms with that. The most eye-opening success of my journey was me realizing that food controlled that way I thought and felt. When I ate healthy home cooked meals that contained fresh ingredients, less sodium and sugar, I made healthier decisions throughout the day; I felt better and the scale finally moved. I absolutely love my wedding pictures. So, all the soon-to-be brides out there, start thinking differently about your lifestyle, workout and eat healthy because wedding pictures won't lie. When you look back at your images you want to love what you see in print."

Broken Heart Meets Fried Chicken

"If you don't take care of this, the most
magnificent machine that you will ever be
given...where are you going to live?"

KARYN CALABRESE

S am hopped off the scale and let out an angry sigh. He was thirty pounds over his comfortable weight. Then he thought of his relationship with Donna. When the relationship was good, it was really good. And, of course when it was bad, it was really bad. What made Sam angry was that good times totally outweighed the bad. He asked himself challenging questions. "Is it possible for me to overlook her inability to commit? I love her so much; maybe I can ignore her psycho ex-boyfriend and his dysfunctional pull on her because of their three children together."

"Nope," he muttered to himself; it's been so long and I've spent so much time waiting. I have to have standards! There's no way that I want this empty, partially committed madness."

Their breakup was difficult to say the least. There was a lot of cursing and yelling. And, even more overindulging in everything else; eating, drinking alcohol, watching tv, listening to angry music and hanging around angry people. This wasn't like him; he was trying to cope. He thought that she should know what to say and do. He felt like she should have the answers, and she just didn't. So to tolerate it all, he sipped more than a few classes of dry Merlot, and overindulged in meat and cheese; and then there was his favorite sweet: carrot cake with a thick decadent cheese cream icing. This spread of indulgent food was a daily late-night occurrence. He felt embarrassed to admit it but he was out of control. In six short months he'd gained thirty pounds, shifted to emotional and spiritual numbness, and had to admit that he was very sad and probably depressed. "I'm tired of this." He gripped the fat around his stomach. "I have to do something." Sam had finally spoken the words that would lead to his journey to freedom and better future self.

Sam gathered the courage to call a friend who was also a trainer. He filled her in on the details of his former relationship and how he had made a turn for the worst but recognized that he had to be pulled back. He said, "I really need help with getting control of my health and weight. I believe that you are the only one who can help in this area. I'll call my therapist to hash out a plan for all the other stuff." His trainer friend agreed and together, they committed to getting Sam back on track.

The first training session was a success. It felt good to be active again. The trainer communicated Sam's plan: to train four times per week for thirty to forty-five minutes, decrease his alcohol intake, and cut out the late-night eating and sleep instead. This wasn't going to be easy—after all, he was still mourning the loss of his love — but he was committed to making a difficult change for his own good. He remained focused and steadfast; he was going to be successful.

It felt like he'd been training for an eternity, but the scale wasn't moving fast enough. "What am I doing wrong?" he asked his trainer. Sam's trainer directed the conversation to his diet. "How much are you eating?" He gave her the run-down. "Monday, Tuesday and Wednesday are great. I'm having stuffed peppers with tofu scramble, onions, and spinach. Lunch is typically a big salad with chickpeas and artichoke hearts. For dinner I like to have tomato basil soup with roasted Brussels sprouts and a hard boiled egg. Thursday, Friday, and Saturday, well those are my cheat days." His cheat foods were things like crispy fried chicken from the fast food chain Popeye's, warm oatmeal raisin cookies with milk, cheesecake, and Merlot. "Okay," the trainer sighed. "Three days of cheating is too much. Please allow yourself one cheat meal twice a week for the next month. Then we will transition you to one cheat meal once per week. You don't have to be perfect, but you need to be consistent."

Sam ate and trained as recommended. In three weeks' time, he'd lost seven pounds. His healthy lifestyle wasn't perfect, but he was focused and committed and that's what mattered most. Sam had learned that overconsumption of all the wrong foods would not make him feel better; it made things worse. He worked on his hurting heart from the inside, and made small, intentional decisions about his food.

If you were to ask Sam today how he made a one-hundred-eighty degree change in his eating habits, he would tell you that he realized that he had to work on overconsumption by healing his heart, not feeding his belly. I heard Sam speaking to another team member; he said, "What I consumed mattered; everyday got easier, and everyday I made the choice to not overdo it."

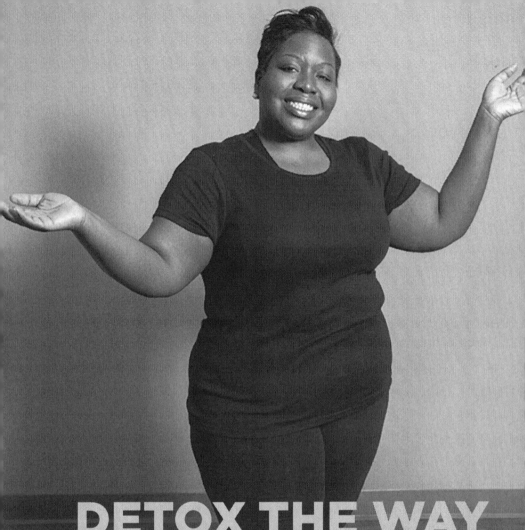

DETOX THE WAY THAT YOU EAT

YOUR COACH'S ADVICE:

There will be days when you feel excited about eating healthy, working out and working on you. There will also be days when you dislike or even hate all of it. Those emotions are normal; feel them, then let them go for they represent only a small moment in time.

Easy doesn't equal the best you. Please don't punk out

Why are you reading this book? Why are you detoxing? What are you aiming to improve? It is important that you be able to answer these questions with clarity if you want to create the best version of yourself. Before we go any further, please pull out your journal and answer the following:

- I am reading this book because:

- I am detoxing because:

- I would like to improve because:

I think you and I can agree that fear, laziness and lack of motivation are all qualities that if allowed, rob us of the opportunity to create the best versions of ourselves, right? They make us "punk out" AKA "give up". I see it happen all the time with my clients. But, I'm here to tell you that I don't want that to happen to you. No more doing the same things over and over hoping for a different result. It's time for you to evolve, and that takes a willingness to be uncomfortable, a lot of effort and some sweat on your part.

What you put into your mind and body matters. The phrase "you are what you eat" is true for the body and the mind. When we feed our minds and bodies junk, the likelihood that we'll have poor mental and physical health increases. And, the opposite is true, when we feed our bodies quality and excellence, then our likely outcome will be quality and excellence. You see, I believe that you have a special purpose in this world, and in order to live it out, you need to grow and evolve in terms of your choices about what you consume.

So, let's start shaping the best you. Your task for this week is to do some cutting in the following areas: overdosing on junk food, junk company, junk television, junk radio, and junk reading. Instead, concentrate on filling yourself with high-quality food, culture, and inspiration and spending time with excellent people.

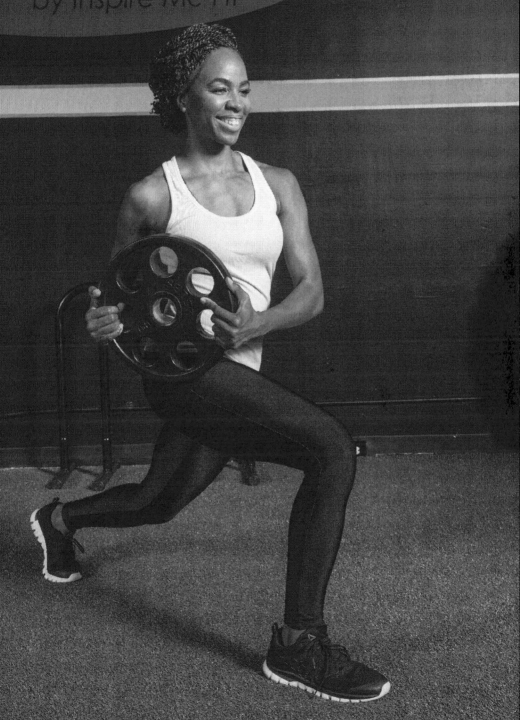

ABOUT YOUR COACH

The desire for wellness comes to us at different times. I became conscious of the term detoxification at the age of nine, when my mother decided that my father had to do one. "Wayne," I remember her saying, "You would have more energy if we eliminated all processed foods from your diet." My father was stubborn, so when mom was able to alter his diet my eyes widened and my hair crinkled. I was intrigued by her persuasive superpowers.

I watched closely as she transformed our frail apartment kitchen into a palace of grand healing. She had no formal training in the science of natural remedies, but she did have the home remedies of the south passed down to her by her mother and grandmother along with a ton of books to guide her gut. My father's harsh reality was a young death but she was on a mission to make every day the best day possible for him.

In her kitchen palace, my mom's loving hands turned nutrient-rich algae into cocoa-flavored puddings, assorted vegetables into rainbow stews, and wheat germ mixtures into "I can't believe it's not meat" entrées. She was the commander and chief of a mission to improve my father's quality of life and by default, we children had to go along for the ride. Today I can see how my unconscious mind decided self-care was the key to living.

YOUR MANTRA

Today and everyday, I choose to listen to
what's going on in my body, mind and spirit.
I promise to love myself enough to respond
when trouble in any of the above surfaces.

But, I'm so busy with the kids

"Respect and honor your Temple – and it will honor you."

SUPANOVA SLOM

Paula looked at herself in the mirror and thought; "I have a family now, I have to work through this". She was a tall, full-figured woman. At five feet ten inches, one hundred eighty pounds, she had come to terms with her caloric needs in comparison to all the other women in her fitness classes. "They're like rabbits," she muttered to herself. "If I tried eating like they eat, I would be weak, hungry and angry." There was no way that she was going back to eating unrealistically. After all, she was a full-figured woman with a full life, so starvation was not an option.

Accepting and allowing herself to eat enough was very logical, but she hadn't figured out how to eat well and still lose weight. Paula evaluated her food journal. "Oh yeah, I had a two protein bars and a peanut butter and jelly sandwich before feeding the kids breakfast.

Gold star for me, I ate really well for breakfast: a homemade chocolate muffin and a vegetable omelet. Lunch has been a little sketchy. I miss my normal salad with grilled chicken a lot of days but I did manage to have a protein bar and my Arizona green tea. Dinner has also been insane. The kids and all of their evening activities have made eating on the go a daily occurrence. Turkey burgers and meatloaf have been my staple proteins, and veggies haven't been so good—sweet potato fries, corn on the cob and sugar snap peas. Well, now that I have the month recorded I can share this information with my fitness trainer. He should be able to offer insight on improvements that will lead to weight loss."

The next day after class Paula privately shared her food log with her trainer. "So, what are your thoughts on that?" Paula asked.

"I think you are a great recorder. Those who keep records typically experience the best results. I also think it's great that you have correlated your food intake with your activities each day. This will help us better understand why you've made certain food choices. A great example of that is when the kids have activities and you have to eat in the car on the go. If weight loss is your goal, let's look to making changes, rather than going on a diet."

"Yeah, I'm tired of starving myself and I'm tired of dieting."

"Great, try this. Prepare your breakfast the night before. We both know that you are a full-figured woman, and you need your nutrients. That will only come from eating fresh, whole foods, including healthy carbohydrates, fats and proteins."

Recommendation number two: when the kids eat breakfast, eat with them but don't over eat by having their food after you've already had a full breakfast. Instead, snack on low sugar fresh fruit, vegetables, or tea. In that way, breakfast time will still feels like a family affair.

Recommendation three: make your lunch to go at the same time that you make lunch for your children. It is highly probable that you will be out running errands, etc., during school hours and won't have time to grab something healthy, so get in the habit of bringing healthy food with you.

Recommendation number four: whenever possible, eat dinner at home. If that doesn't work, choose your top five healthy restaurants that you are confident will offer you and your children high-quality healthy food options. When that is not possible, and you need to eat in the car or at practice, include healthy easy to eat finger foods like hummus and veggies, cup of homemade soup, organic cage free hard boiled eggs, meatballs and/or steak strips.

Recommendation number five: cut down significantly on your packaged snack foods. Plan to eat healthy real food all the time. That includes breakfast, lunch, dinner, and snack time. Instead of bags of popcorn and a protein bar, have hummus and vegetables, piece or cup of fresh fruit and nuts or nut butter or a whole ripe avocado.

Recommendation number six: when eating, ask yourself if the food that you are about to consume are nutrient-rich or nutrient-poor. Chances are, if it's deep fried, bagged, canned or boxed, or lives in the frozen section, it is probably nutrient-weak. Try to eat raw fruits and vegetables several times daily.

"Wow, that's a lot."

"I know, Paula, it can be but do this: introduce only one action item per week. If it works for a week, chances are that it will fit into your life. If it doesn't, we'll know right away. If any of your lifestyle changes start to feel overwhelming, simply shift the change to something that feels more manageable and I can help with that."

"I think I can work with that."

After two months of consistency and hard work Paula dropped eleven pounds. She was grateful that she had finally gotten advice that worked.

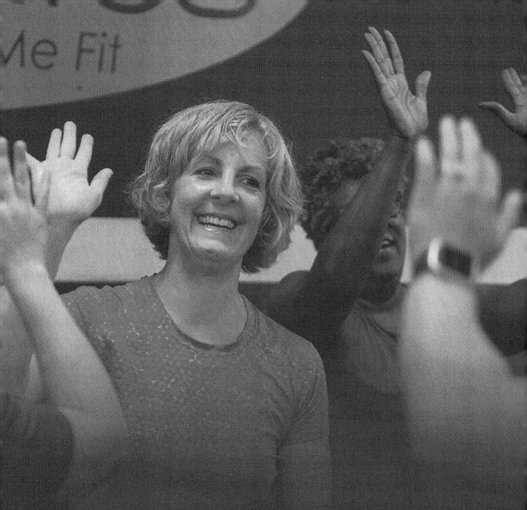

DETOX THE WAY THAT YOU EAT

YOUR COACH'S ADVICE:

It is very likely that the change you want will not be instant. Plan to keep calm, lean into the work, stay connected to your team and the results you want will come.

LIVE LIFE TOOL

Learn to be still. Once per week, spend thirty minutes alone with the intentions of processing where you are in your life and what you're doing. Reflect on the ups and downs of the week. Once per month, spend one hour alone reflecting on the month. Once per quarter, spend a weekend alone contemplating and reflecting on your life. Once per year take a full week with yourself. Take time to plan for an even better you.

What's wrong with my diet?

*"Because we cannot scrub our inner body, we need
to learn a few skills to help cleanse our tissues,
organs, and mind. This is the art of Ayurveda."*

SEBASTIAN POLE

"I don't know what it is or what I need to do. I train hard. I eat fairly healthy. I drink water. But I just can't get rid of this bulge in my lower stomach. Look at this; you can pinch more than an inch." It was clear that Jina was frustrated. She was on her last set of burpees, but was focused on what was wrong with her body. Her trainer wanted her to focus on how strong and powerful she was.

Jina's trainer complimented her. "Let me first say how amazing and strong you were during your workout today, great job." Jina looked annoyed and didn't respond. "If the goal is for you to tone up your midsection we will need to do that in three ways: address the fat around the belly via your diet, reduce bloat and build muscle; you will need to improve your water intake daily, more abdominal work on your off days as well as exercises that focus on increasing your intensity."

Jina still looked frustrated. "Seriously, I've been working at this for over 6 months and I'm still not where I want to be. I'm 185 pounds now and my goal is to be 175. My waist is 35 inches and I want it to be 30. I'm not a fat woman, but I do have goals, and I need to know if you can help me."

Jina's trainer understood where she was coming from, and she could even understand why she was frustrated.

"What I want you to keep in mind is that you have strong abdominal muscles. What we are trying to address is the fat that is smothering the muscles. You also have a bit of bloating in your lower abdominals, and the reason I know its bloating is because the bulge isn't always the same from session to session. Some sessions it's bigger than others." Look, the reality is that we are in our forties and hormonally our bodies are changing. But, while it is much more challenging to lose belly fat when hormonal changes happen, it is NOT IMPOSSIBLE!

Jina looked relieved. She felt like her trainer was making sense.

"Okay I can see that," Jina responded. "So what do we do about that fat and the bloat?"

"Easy," the trainer replied. "We increase your water intake to 80 ounces per day and we modify your diet, so that you're consuming more high in fiber plants, lean protein, and low to no starch. Your proteins are going to build and repair your muscles. Reducing your starch and pushing your workouts will help us use of some of your fat storage. Increasing your fiber with dark green leafy vegetables will help to push waste through the large intestine, as well as reduce the appearance of bloat and flatten your lower abs. You also need to work with your gynecologist to establish a plan of action for testing and maintaining healthy hormone levels."

"Okay, I think I can handle that but sticking to the new food plan may be difficult and will likely need some adjusting". Jina was an executive in a busy corporation, so there were many times that she worked through breakfast and lunch, only leaving time for a protein bar and yogurt. Jina knew that although her grab and go foods contain protein, they were considered snack foods and that was not what her trainer was suggesting for meals. Jina's trainer had explained that she wanted Jina to eat three to four ounces of lean protein, no more than a quarter of a cup of starchy foods, and three to four cups of vegetables, 50 percent of them being raw and 50 percent cooked. This was supposed to happen for two of her three meals daily.

Jina's first week of trying to adopt this new regimen was a bust. She just couldn't find the time to prepare the foods or eat them. Jina went back to her trainer. "Here's what's happening," Jina explained. "I could totally eat what you recommended, but those foods are not convenient and I need convenience."

Jina's trainer smiled. "Jina, of course we can make this grab and go. Here's a list of high fiber, lean protein grab and go breakfast, lunch and dinner options. Use this pen and circle the ones you would most likely adopt." Jina read out the meals from the list that sounded good to her, "broccoli omelet muffins, tomatoes basil soup, open face black bean burger, avocado and tomato lettuce wraps."

Jina's trainer said, "Those sound like great options. Please watch your portions and include a salad as often as you can with each of the dishes."

Jina tried the food plan again, and by the end of the week, she couldn't believe how amazing she felt. She was not only able to keep to the plan, but her belly had flattened, she had tons of energy and felt strong. It took Jina two months before she saw the fat loss she wanted in her lower abs. But after eight months of training, she was glad that she and her trainer had found a solution.

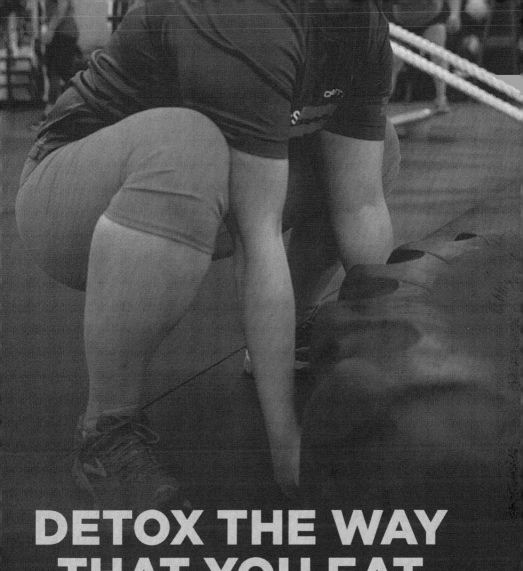

DETOX THE WAY THAT YOU EAT

YOUR COACH'S ADVICE:

Be both honest and brave when it comes to why your current circumstances are what they are; then decide to address the problem by finding a solution that allows you to reconcile the situation.

It's my medication, isn't it

"Mindful eating is about eating with awareness. When you eat mindfully, you slow down, pay attention to the food you are eating, and savor every bite."

SUSAN ALBERS

"The scale hasn't budged in two months. I think that I've hit a plateau." "What's wrong, have you changed your diet at all?" Tina asked."I'm not sure, but I can tell you that I don't eat that much. As a matter of fact, I'm only eating two meals per day tops. When I drink my coffee, it's black, and I very rarely eat junk food. Maybe ice cream every now and again but nothing major. I think that the scale should be moving. After all, I'm working out with my trainer twice a week. I take boot camp five days a week, and I'm hardly eating."

A group of Jill's girlfriends from the gym were now gathered in a circle discussing Jill's lack of results.

"Jill, have you had a heart-to-heart talk with your trainer? Part of their job is to help you see results."

"I have," Jill replied, "but I wasn't really happy with her response."

"Well, what did she say?"

"She said that my diet needs changing, but honestly, after my last session I checked out of our conversation and stopped listening to her because I feel like, 'there is no way that I can eat less than what I am eating right now.'"

"But Jill," Barbara used an encouraging tone. "Maybe this isn't about eating less; maybe it's about eating differently. What if you gave the conversation with your trainer a fair chance? You might see changes." Jill considered what Barbara and the rest of the group were saying.

"Maybe you're right about having another heart-to-heart with my trainer. I'll bring up my frustration with not seeing results, and I'll give her advice some serious consideration because I am determined to get this weight off of me."

Jill's next session was on a Wednesday morning. Her trainer asked her to pop on the scale. "You see! The scale is not moving."

"Jill," her trainer sighed. "Let's get your workout in first then we can discuss how to get your numbers moving in the right direction."

"That's fine," Jill replied. Twenty-five minutes had passed quickly, and Jill was thoroughly exhausted, but she collected her thoughts and the last bit of energy she had so that she could be present in the conversation.

Jill began the conversation. "I'm fat and I'm never going to lose this weight. Everyone in my family is thin, but me, I look horrible. I am doing everything right. I am doing everything to the best of my ability. My doctor told me that the medications that I'm taking are causing my numbers to stall; there is no way that I can stop taking my medicine." She was clearly frustrated. Jill's trainer stopped her. "Jill, I really need you to listen to what I am about to say. The challenge of the scale not moving could definitely be the medication that you are taking as well as having high stress, lack of sleep and certain allergies to foods. But we have to start somewhere, so let's begin by making a few diet modifications. That will only help improve the likelihood of you getting positive results."

Jill blurted out, "I knew you were going to say that".

"Well, it is. Okay, first things first, let's go to the pharmacy across the street where you get your prescriptions filled. I'd like for you to talk with your pharmacist about the effects of the medications that you are taking. Then your job is to call your doctor and discuss what the pharmacist shared with you as well as the potential for food allergies, high stress and lack of sleep as reasons for the scale not moving. "Sounds good," Jill replied.

"Now as it relates to your diet, I have a few questions. Please answer as honestly as possible: how many times a day are you eating?" Jill responded, "Let's go through your questions first."

"I typically eat one to two times per day."

"What are you eating?"

"I am eating fowl, you know, chicken, turkey, sometimes fish and very rarely beef. I'll have that with grits or eggs if it's breakfast. If it's lunch or dinner I'll eat a baked sweet potato."

"I'm just curious; do any of those meals contain vegetables?"

"Yes, corn or canned string beans. I don't like to buy fresh food because it's just me in the house and that stuff goes bad too quickly."

Jill's trainer took notes. "I see," she said. "How is your water intake?"

"I drink water a couple of times of day; I think I consume one to two sixteen ounce water bottles per day."

"Great, do you have any idea how much refined sugar, sodium, and fat you consume?"

"Not really," Jill said.

"One last question before I make some recommendations that are going to help you burn a lot of fat and move the scale. What time of day are you eating your first and last meal?"

Jill replied, "Sometimes around noon for my first meal and around 8 or 9 o'clock for my last."

"Thank you, Jill; I really appreciate your honesty. I'm 100 percent sure if we make a few small changes like you sharing your journey with your doctor and you taking their recommendations seriously as well as you making a few diet modifications, you will see positive fat loss results."

"Well, tell me what they are," Jill said with excitement.

"To see the scale move, you do need to eat regularly, so if you're up by 6am and training by 8 am you should really try to eat something small at least one hour before your training, or by 10am once all your training is done. Eating more regularly will help your body realize that it is not being starved and will improve your potential for fat burning. Please keep in mind that when you're asleep, you're actually fasting. So all of your body systems slow down, and when you wake up you come out of your fasting state, and to jumpstart your metabolism you do need to eat or drink something or your body will remain sluggish until you eat or drink. Once we find a morning eating time that works, the goal is to be consistent with that eating time so that your body expects that input. You don't have to consume a lot but should consume something."

"Now, let's talk about food options. In general aim to keep your refined sugar intake low. Examples of where you might see refined sugar are yogurts, beverages, jarred sauces, some meats, most snack foods, candies, cookies, pastries, ice creams, etc. Allow yourself only 24 grams of refined sugar daily. To give you a gauge of what 24 grams is, use a single serving of yogurt. It typically contains sixteen to twenty-six grams of sugar which means that you would only have one serving of yogurt and meet your quota for the day. Like sugar, sodium is in everything. Sodium is added to a lot of packaged foods because it can act as a preservative and it also adds flavor. But we need to be careful about how much we consume because overconsumption can cause serious health problems."

"Here's something to keep in mind. One system of the body is called the endocrine system. Within that system are our kidneys. The kidneys function to clean the blood in order to create urine and remove the waste from our bodies. We help our kidneys to function well when we drink water. Any nephrologists or kidney doctor will tell you to use your urine as a testament of whether or not you're drinking enough water. If your urine is pale yellow to clear, then you are taking in enough. If your urine is dark yellow and has a scent then you're not taking in enough. What I would say is, if you can drink half your body weight in ounces you would be ahead of the game. For example, if someone weighs 140 pounds they would consume 70 ounces of water."

"Now, let's talk about how much you should be eating. If we were going to just eyeball your food, your meat should fit in the palm of your hand. Your starches should fit without spilling out in the cup of your hand. Those two items make up half of your nine-inch plate. The other half is vegetables. 50 percent of your vegetables should be raw and the other 50 percent should be cooked. To be more precise, we could weigh your food and your meat would be three to four ounces per serving no more than twice per day. Your starch would be one quarter to half a cup cooked no more than twice per day and you'd have four to six cups of vegetables per day."

"All that sounds good," Jill said, "but what if I want something sweet or salty? Like a dessert or popcorn during a movie."

"Those are very good questions. There's nothing wrong with eating dessert or having a salty snack. But I would like for us to shift our mindset so that snacks are real food. By that I mean; we are moving away from poor-quality food that has no vitamins or minerals, we are moving closer to foods that have lots of vitamins and minerals. So, when you're looking for a snack, don't grab your bag of chips— instead, grab your homemade applesauce, sliced cucumbers and hummus or your okra popcorn. All of those foods have the vitamins and minerals that we need to feel satisfied. They are all what we call nutrient-dense foods. So if you want something sweet, let's aim for nature's sweet foods, like fruits. If you want something salty, the approach is the same."

"Here's a sample menu, and take a look at this list of foods to avoid and foods to embrace. As you can see, 80 percent of the time you need to eat really healthy, 20 percent of the time if you're not perfect, you'll still see positive fat loss."

Jill collected the documents. "Great, now let's head to the pharmacy to find out about my medication." The pharmacist confirmed that two out of the five medications that Jill was taking was known to cause weight gain. She recommended that Jill talk with her doctor about alternative brands of the same drugs that would not cause weight gain as well as adjusting her dosage. Jill took the recommendations back to her doctor and was able to have the dosage of one medication adjusted and the other swapped out for a generic brand of the same drug.

Additionally, Jill reluctantly adopted the menu that her trainer recommended almost out of spite. She didn't really believe she would see positive fat loss results! But 30 days later, Jill was down seven and a half pounds.

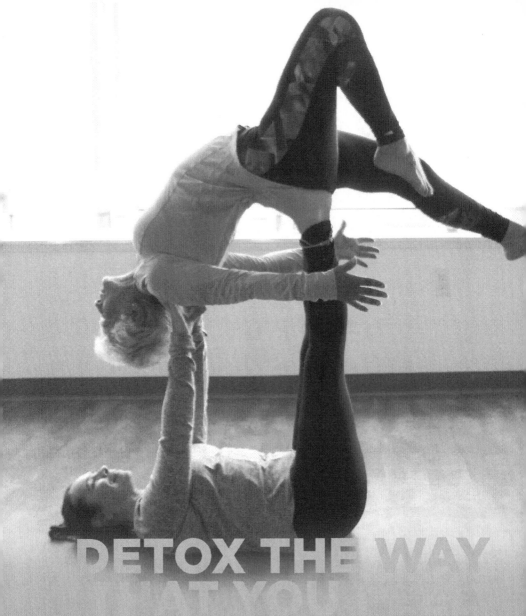

DETOX THE WAY

YOUR COACH'S ADVICE:

Extreme behaviors on either side of the spectrum—overeating or overly restricting what you eat—are not sustainable or healthy. Look for personal balance whenever you can.

LIVE LIFE TOOL

Music! Allow this playlist to motivate you.

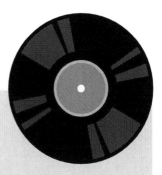

EAT IT PLAYLIST

- **I'm A Survivor** by Destiny's Child
- **Should I Stay Or Should I Go** by The Clash
- **The Climb** by Miley Cirus
- **Life Changes** by Thomas Rhett
- **Better Together** by Jack Johnson
- **Activity Idle Breeze and Its Recipes** by Flitz & Suppe
- **Thunder** by Imagine Dragons
- **Eye Of The Tiger** by Survivor Rocky IV
- **Not Afraid** by Eminem
- **Best OF You** by Foo Fighters

FITNESS TRAINING TIPS

Whoo hoo! You made it through 2 full weeks of activity. Great job! Continue to pace yourself appropriately; modify your regimen when needed, and maintain your mix of cardiovascular, strength, mobility and flexibility training weekly.

EAT IT!

Week Two

WORKOUT FOR DETOXIFICATION

LET YOUR WARM-UP BEGIN!

- Hit this workout at least **four times this week**. We have begun the process of training your thoughts, and now we need to train to be more disciplined. One way that we will begin developing discipline is by changing some behaviors that are typically a result of stress, such as overeating or making poor food choices. **No longer will you eat your stress**. Instead, you'll exercise your stress away.

- Do each movement for 30 – 60 seconds and repeat it two to three times before beginning your strength work. Take your time, make your moves as big as possible, and go at a slow to medium pace.

ALTERNATING SPINAL BALANCE

- Keep your arms fully extended, as if you're pushing the floor down

- Maintain a flat back while engaging your abs

- Fully extend your arms and legs

- Be sure to keep your hips rotating downward

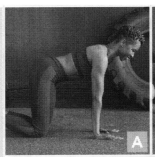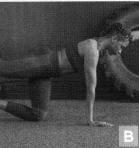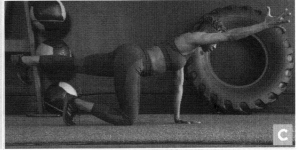

SINGLE SIDE CLAM SHELL

- Bring your arms slightly wider than shoulder-width apart

- Raise your leg out to the side, like a door opening and closing

- Avoid leaning to one side. Do your best to stay in the middle

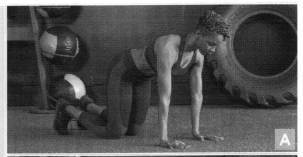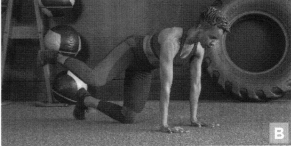

MOUNTAIN CLIMBERS

- Bring your body into a plank

- Either tap or jump alternating legs forward

- Aim to pull the leg between your arms towards your nose

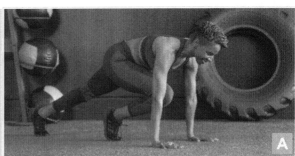

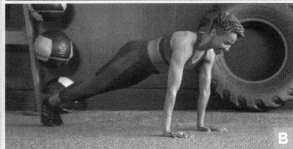

GREAT JOB!

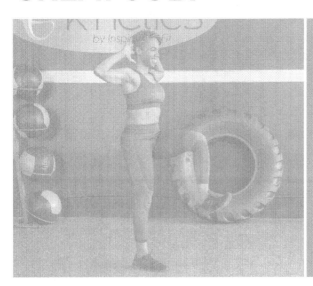

TIP OF THE DAY

You will achieve the best results by making sure that you are appropriately challenged. Too little of the right effort will stall your improvements; too much of the wrong effort will likely compromise proper form and cause preventable injury.

Take your time! If you need assistance all you have to do is reach out.

STRENGTH WORKOUT

COMPLETE EXERCISES AS FOLLOWS:

- 30 seconds of work for beginners with a maximum of 60 seconds of rest between exercises

- 60 seconds of work for intermediate to advanced exercisers with no more than 30 seconds of rest between exercises

- 60 seconds of work for advanced exercisers with no rest between exercises

- Go in this order: leg, push, hinge, pull exercises; Complete two to four sets

- Complete one to two sets of cool-down exercises once your strength work is done

LEG EXERCISES

WALKING LUNGES

- For every lunge, add a torso rotation

- Twist towards your bent knee

- If you're feeling off-balance, it is okay for you to step a little wider in your stance

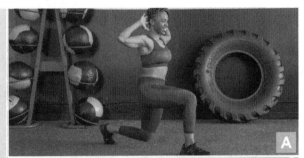
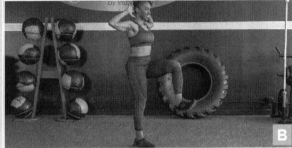

HALF VICTORY SQUATS

- Bring your hands behind your head

- Keep your chest up as you squat

- Sit as low as you can in your squat. Aim for your hamstrings to be parallel to the floor

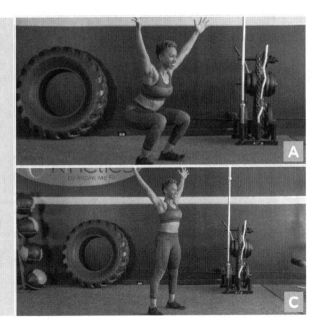

LATERAL LEG RAISES

- Carry out this movement from either standing tall or with bent knees

- Raise your leg out to the side without rotating your hip upward

- Add more challenge by adding a step for height variation

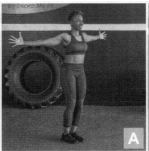 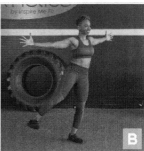 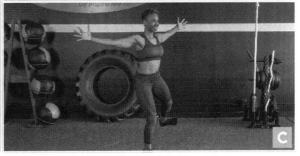

PUSH EXERCISES

OVERHEAD TRICEP EXTENSION WITH A RESISTANCE BAND

- From a kneeling position, take the band behind your back

- Holding the band with both hands, extend the band fully

- Engage your abs to avoid arching your back

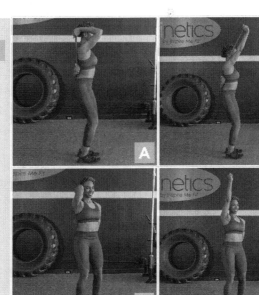

STAGGERED PUSH-UP

- This push-up variation can be done off the wall, a bench or the floor

- Remember that one hand should replace the other for each push up

- Drop your knees to make the movement a little easier

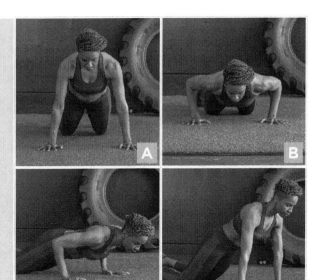

HINGE EXERCISES

LOW OR HIGH IMPACT SQUAT THRUST

- Begin this movement from a standing position

- Place your hands on a sturdy surface

- Step or hop back to plank, stand and repeat

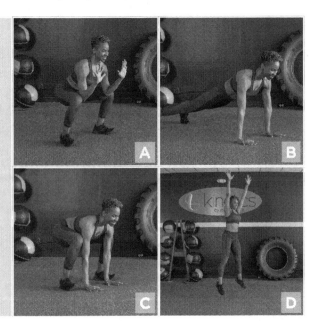

JERSEY TWISTS

- Bring yourself to a seated position

- Be sure that you aren't sitting into your low back

- Engage your lower abs

- Rotate as far right and left as you can

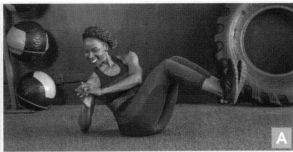

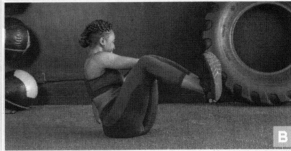

SUPINE DOUBLE LEG UP

- From a seated position, bring your arms much wider than your body

- Lift your legs together, rotating them from one side to the other

- Place a prop on the floor to act as a marker to lift your legs up and over

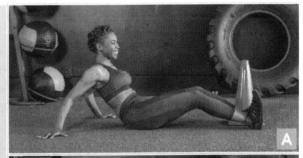

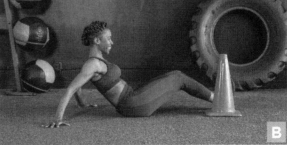

SUPINE HORIZONTAL SCISSOR KICKS

- Lay flat on your back and tuck flat palms underneath your bottom

- Bring knees into the chest then extend them

- Horizontally kick keeping the low back on the floor

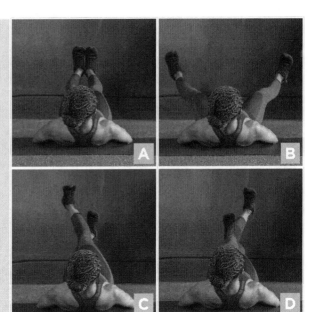

PULLS EXERCISES

WALL SIT "T" OUT

- From your wall sit, extend your arms away from your body

- Extend your arms fully, making the letter "T"

- Be sure to keep tension in your band the entire time

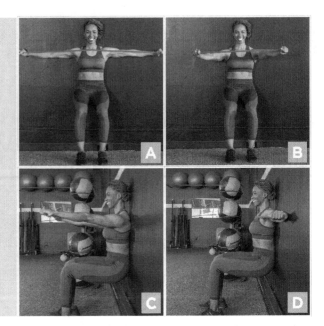

STATIONARY LUNGE UPWARD PULL

- Come into a lunge position with the band underneath one of your feet

- With your arms straight, lift them towards the ceiling without bending your elbows

- Engage your abs to avoid arching your back

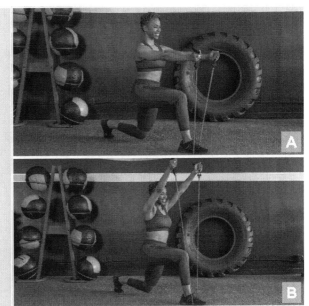

KNEELING DIAGONAL PULL

- Kneel, and bring your arms to clam position

- Be sure to get the appropriate tension in the band. You should be able to extend your arms fully

- Engage your abs to avoid arching your back

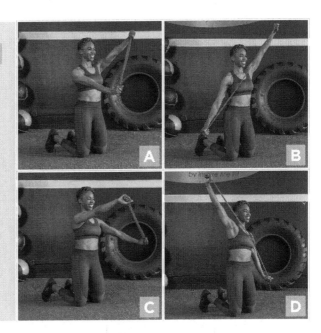

COOL-DOWN STRETCHES

STANDING SINGLE ARM CROSS OVER

- Stand tall with your arms long in "T" position

- Draw one arm across your body

- Use the opposite arm to comfortably stretch the arm that is fully extended

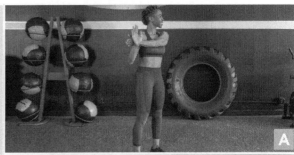

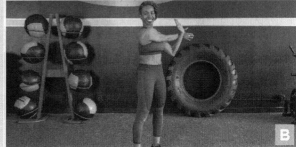

STANDING YOGA "4"

- Do this free standing or holding onto a wall

- Bring one ankle to cross over your low leg or thigh

- If you are able to get the ankle to your thigh, attempt to sit down as if you are sitting in a chair

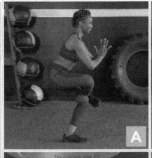
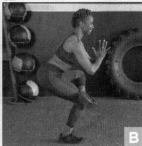
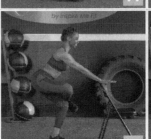
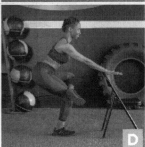

TRICEP SIDE BODY STRETCH

- From a full stand, reach your arm behind yourself, as if you're patting yourself on the back

- With your opposite hand, comfortably push your elbow to increase the stretch in the back of your arm

- Take a side bend, stretching away from the bent elbow

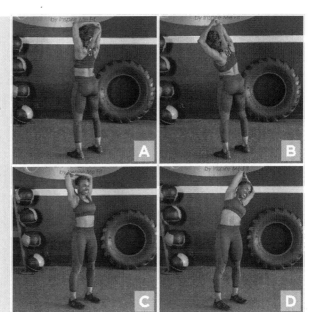

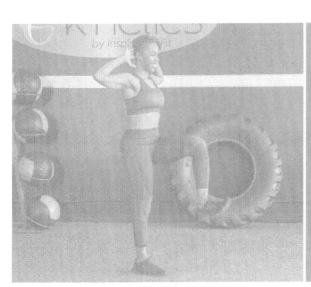

TIP OF THE DAY

Be mindful that if you feel an usual amount of muscular fatigue or muscular cramping it may be because you are dehydrated.

DO drink an adequate amount of water prior to working out.

7 DAY READ IT AND EAT IT SAMPLE MENU FOR DETOXIFICATION

DAY 1

Pre-breakfast: 8 ounce glass of lemon or lime water, either warm or room temperature

Breakfast: protein drink of your choice with your choice of decaf coffee or tea

Lunch: vegetarian stuffed cabbage with your choice of side salad

Dinner: cream of spinach with your choice of side salad

Snack options: sliced raw vegetables (avoid sweet vegetables like carrots or beets this week) and/or one serving of any non-sweet snack found in the snack recipes section. To achieve the best fat loss results, limit snack foods to 200 calories or less. Do your best to consume 64-80 ounces of water today while keeping your sodium intake to 2,000mg total or less.

DAY 2

Pre-breakfast: 8 ounce glass of lemon or lime water, either warm or room temperature

Breakfast: quarter of a cup wake'em up oats, fresh fruit with your choice of decaf coffee or tea

Lunch: no-bread black bean burger or salmon patty with steamed cauliflower rice and your choice of side salad

Dinner: vegetable broth with a your choice of salad

Snack options: sliced raw vegetables (avoid sweet vegetables like carrots or beets this week) and/or one serving of any non-sweet snack found in the snack recipes section. To achieve the best fat loss results, limit snack foods to 200 calories or less. Do your best to consume 64-80 ounces of water today while keeping your sodium intake to 2,000mg total or less.

DAY 3

Pre-breakfast: 8 ounce glass of lemon or lime water, either warm or room temperature

Breakfast: protein drink of your choice, and your choice of decaf coffee or tea

Lunch: cream of mushroom sauce with zoodles, and your choice of side salad

Dinner: sweet potato crumb soup with your choice of side salad

Snack options: sliced raw vegetables (avoid sweet vegetables like carrots or beets this week) and/or one serving of any non-sweet snack found in the snack recipes section. To achieve the best fat loss results, limit snack foods to 200 calories or less. Do your best to consume 64-80 ounces of water today while keeping your sodium intake to 2,000mg total or less.

DAY 4

Pre-breakfast: 8 ounce glass of lemon or lime water, either warm or room temperature

Breakfast: omelet of your choice, mixed greens and your choice of decaf coffee or tea

Lunch: non-dairy spinach lasagna with your choice of side salad

Dinner: hearty lentil soup with your choice of side salad

Snack options: sliced raw vegetables (avoid sweet vegetables like carrots or beets this week) and/or one serving of any non-sweet snack found in the snack recipes section. To achieve the best fat loss results, limit snack foods to 200 calories or less. Do your best to consume

64-80 ounces of water today while keeping your sodium intake to 2,000mg total or less.

DAY 5

Pre-breakfast: 8 ounce glass of lemon or lime water, either warm or room temperature

Breakfast: quarter of a cup of cream of quinoa, fresh fruit and your choice decaf coffee or tea

Lunch: Greek salad with grilled tofu, fish or seitan

Dinner: chunky cream of salmon or black bean soup with your choice of side salad

Snack options: sliced raw vegetables (avoid sweet vegetables like carrots or beets this week) and/or one serving of any non-sweet snack found in the snack recipes section. To achieve the best fat loss results, limit snack foods to 200 calories or less. Do your best to consume 64-80 ounces of water today while keeping your sodium intake to 2,000mg total or less.

DAY 6

Pre-breakfast: 8 ounce glass of lemon or lime water, either warm or room temperature

Breakfast: protein drink of choice

Lunch: sautéed fresh vegetables over cauliflower rice

Dinner: carrot ginger soup, the recommended serving amount of flax crackers, and your choice of side salad

Snack options: sliced raw vegetables (avoid sweet vegetables like carrots or beets this week) and/or one serving of any non-sweet snack found in the snack recipes section. To achieve the best fat loss results, limit snack foods to 200 calories or less. Do your best to consume 64-80 ounces of water today while keeping your sodium intake to 2,000mg total or less.

DAY 7

Pre-breakfast: 8 ounce glass of lemon or lime water, either warm or room temperature

Breakfast: quarter of a cup wake'um up oats, fresh fruit and your choice of decaf coffee or tea

Lunch: sautéed zoodles and stewed curry vegetables with your choice of side salad

Dinner: Jenny's Creamy Split Pea Soup with your choice of side salad

Snack options: sliced raw vegetables (avoid sweet vegetables like carrots or beets this week) and/or one serving of any non-sweet snack found in the snack recipes section. To achieve the best fat loss results, limit snack foods to 200 calories or less. Do your best to consume 64-80 ounces of water today while keeping your sodium intake to 2,000mg total or less.

In week three we'll carry over the positive changes we've made in how we think and what we consume, and extend them to working to improve how we feel. This week, there is typically a lot of emotional purging that must happen. Pick your favorite quote and post it where it can be seen often.

FEEL IT!

EMOTIONAL DETOXIFICATION

Desperate for change

"With the new day comes new strength and new thoughts."

ELEANOR ROOSEVELT

She was tall with long limbs and a narrow waist. She had no concerns about body fat percentages, efforts to slim down or tone up. Nope, her concerns were that she was fifty-five, physically stiff, easily winded, low energy, recently divorced and lacked the motivation to make improvements.

"I am out of shape," she explained. "That's why I need your help. I just can't find the energy to get it done on my own." I let out an empathetic sigh. "Let's do this. Let's not make your desire to be in better shape rational. You're an intelligent woman and I know that you know what to do. Instead, let's get your emotions stirred about it. It is from an emotional place that we will make long lasting improvements."

She nodded a hesitant yes. "Why do you want to be in better shape? Let's say I snap my fingers and you are instantly in your ideal shape; how will your life improve?" There was a long silence between us. Her eyes filled with tears. "You want the truth? Well, here it is! I'm getting old. I feel my age and I don't like it. I'm divorced and feeling alone. I want to remarry. I want a life partner." More tears fell from her eyes. "I want to make a change. I have to make a change. My children are older. They don't need me the way that they use to. This has to get better."

I smiled a comforting smile. "I want you to hold on to those feelings because those emotions will:

- Make you show up for every push-up, squat and lunge

- Hit the recommended ten thousand cardio steps daily

- Inspire you to eat less sugar and drink more water

"Most of us make improvements when we are emotionally stirred. I'm excited about your journey towards better health and wellness. This positive paradigm shift will stir your physical, mental, emotional and spiritual self for the good." We shared a smile. "High-five to you; let's soar!"

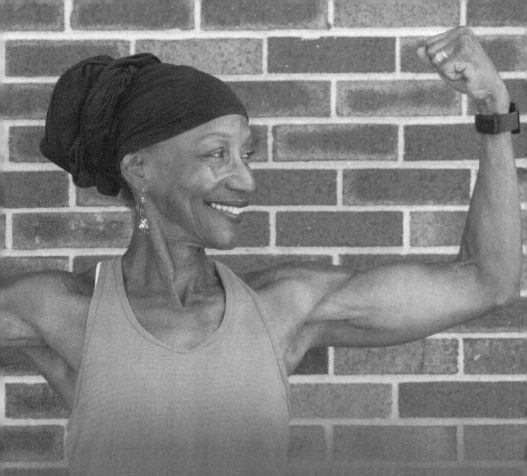

DETOX THE WAY THAT YOU LIVE

YOUR COACH'S ADVICE:

A wise elder once told me and I believe that it is true; In order for you to create the very best version of yourself including you having better fitness, fat loss and enhanced energy you must marry the vision of you that lives in your head with the vision of you that lives in your heart. When those two things live in harmony, longevity of a better you will also exist.

Something good came out of it

"You have power over your mind – not outside events. Realize this and you will find strength."

MARCUS AURELIUS

Her belly button had literally changed positions. It no longer faced the floor, weighed down by gravity and fat. Now it faced forward, and was sunken in, just the way she liked it. The length of her arms had changed as well. They no longer stopped above her waist. Now the palms of her hands reached mid-thigh, a look that she loved because it meant that she had less fat around her back. Maya smiled and said, "These changes are nothing short of a miracle. I have spent my entire life in this suit and this suit is changing right before my eyes."

Maya loved her mother, but this problem with her weight was partially her mother's fault. Maya spoke again. "My mother has a very negative self-image. I look like her, and so she also has a negative image of me. From the time I was nine, she insisted that I diet. She told me that being pudgy looked bad and was not ladylike. To a young, impressionable girl, if your mother thinks you're ugly, well then, you must be ugly. When I was fifteen, her insults got worse. She said no boy would ever take a girl like me to the prom; I would be heavier than he was and that would be disgusting. When I was twenty-eight, she told me that marriage would never happen for a girl like me with a double gut and double chin. It was all horrible to hear and it totally robbed me of my self-esteem."

"Oh my, so how did you work through the challenge of self hate?"

"I don't think that I have," Maya replied. "I think that every day, I wake up and I decide to love and accept myself. Now don't get me wrong, I have come a long way with learning how to think positively about myself. And, most of my improvements have come because I started working on all the things that I felt were wrong with me. My weight was always a problem, so I started working out, and because of it I am physically, mentally, and emotionally transforming for the better. And, every day it takes work not to let that quiet voice inside of my head tell me that I am worthless, disgusting, ugly, fat, not the marrying type and more."

Maya's "Live Life for a New You" support group listened to her intently. "Honestly, all I needed was to see that something that I was doing was right; that there was something, anything good that could come from me. I started my weight-loss journey and couldn't believe that I was losing weight. Something that I was doing was actually working, and seeing that I could make changes has inspired me to keep going. I constantly work to keep my mother and every other negative person or thing that tries to attack me at bay. This allows me to focus on making a better me every second of every day. You all inspire me as well; my fitness family. You motivate me and keep me reaching for more. I actually have a team of people to help to keep me focused, and it is from that place that I stay lifted and excited about how awesome my life is becoming daily. I realized that it is all my choice."

LIVE LIFE TOOL

Words have the power to reshape the way you feel, think and respond. Read and listen to inspiring books or audiobooks as often as possible and allow your positive reprogramming to begin.

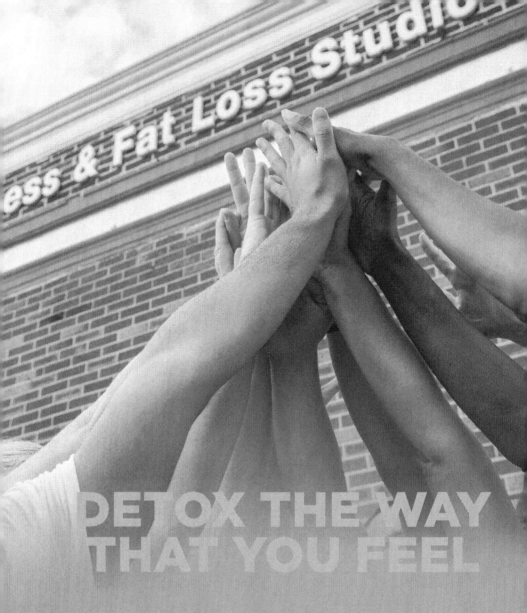

DETOX THE WAY THAT YOU FEEL

YOUR COACH'S ADVICE:

Life feels like less of a burden when we use our family, friends and community to help us cope during the rough patches of our lives. Seek out positive and uplifting company to help keep you lifted; and, never be afraid to ask for help. It is a sign of strength.

Overcoming the pull

*"Every form of addiction is bad, no matter whether
the narcotic be alcohol or morphine or idealism."*

CARL JUNG

For the first time in a long time, Bill felt alive. Friends and family members complimented him on taking ownership of his life. He admitted that the pain that he felt existed on every level. It was physical, emotional, and mental. At some point life had gotten so bad that Bill could feel his sorrow deep inside of his bones. He could feel frustration and worry circulating through his bloodstream. The last five years had just about killed him. But he was finally starting to see the light of day. For the first time in a long time, life was letting up and he could breathe again.

"Not many people recover from this sort of trauma," whispered Freeda, his therapist. "You are doing a remarkable job." Bill had hit rock bottom after losing his job of twenty years, his wife, his children, his parents and all of his self respect. In five years, he had managed to lose everything worth anything to him. His addictions had spun out of control and he had nothing. Bill no longer cried out, he used heroin and drank. He no longer spoke with friends for support; when he ate, his diet was junk and drugs. He went on like this for what seemed like an eternity. He had no hope and no longer cared about anything or anyone.

"What is marvelous, Bill, is that even at your lowest point you managed to see signs that your life is not over and that the world still needs and wants you." It was sort of a miracle, how it happened. One day, in a high and drunken state, Bill had bumped into an old girlfriend. She had known Bill to be a very successful business man and was surprised to see how low he had sunk. Bill's ex passed him her business card, and on the back were the words, "Your life is not over. You can come back from this." It would take Bill weeks of holding on to the card, thinking about the card, and carrying the card before he actually had the strength to call his friend. After he finally did, his life was never the same. What Bill didn't know at the time was that his ex was also a recovering addict who had become an addiction counselor and therapist. She had transformed her life, and had made it her life's mission to help others do the same thing. Bill spoke to his friend every day, sometimes twice a day, for a month before following through and checking himself into a rehab facility. The strength Bill got from going into alcohol and drug rehab gave him the strength to seek out a spiritual center for practice. With spiritual practice came a deep love and gratitude for life and living. Bill made a decision to live. With a lot of prayer, discipline and effort he stopped drinking and getting high. He was eating healthy. He was exercising. Bill removed everything and everyone in his life that he felt brought him to a dark place. He replaced those things and people with things that brought him joy. His life has never been the same.

"Bill," Freeda spoke. "Your freedom journey will always be a journey. It is something that you will work on for the rest of your life. But as you can see, you have the power and ability to win in every way possible. Do you believe what I am saying to you?"

"Yes!" Bill replied

"Do you know that you are a winner?"

"Yes!" Bill replied.

"Do you realize that you are part of a great universe and that your contribution to society matters?'

"Yes!" Bill replied.

'Say the words then, Bill. Tell me what you know is the truth about yourself."

"I am a blissful and whole being. I have a lot to give to this world. I am happy and whole today and every day because I choose to be. Today and every day I choose to live the fullest, happiest life that I can possibly live."

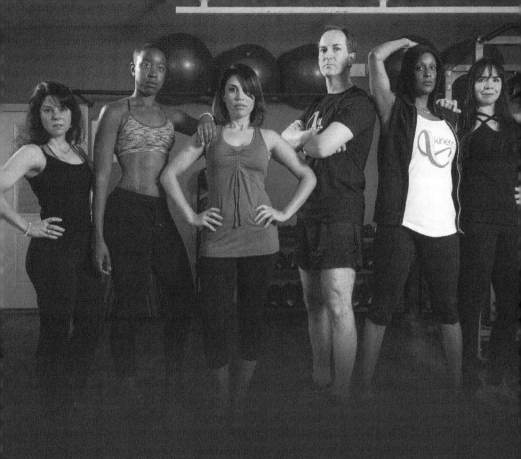

DETOX THE WAY THAT YOU FEEL

YOUR COACH'S ADVICE:

Negativity is all around us, so when you find your tribe, keep them close; they will help build your confidence, keep you steadfast and strong.

Ugh! I hate all of this but I love the results

"Clarity of thought and action is key"

METRA LUNDY

It's so much easier to eat chocolate chip pancakes. Ugh! I hate all of this. The food restrictions; the sweating; the happy go lucky push-up loving people I that are all around me; oh, and the reality that if I want to maintain this level of fitness and my current physique that I will need to commit to doing this for the rest of my life.

I glanced back with a blank stare. Yep, I get it. Are you clear about what foods to eat this week and which ones to avoid? You're puffy and your ankles are a warning sign that something is off in your body and we need to respond. Let's adjust your diet as well as your workout. Coach, I heard you; I know what foods to eat and the ones to avoid. Great; are you clear about your training schedule for this week as well as your challenge exercises? It's important that we meet our four day minimum. Yes, I have that down as well. Cool; last but definitely not the least, are you good to go with the reading and journaling work that I asked you to complete? I am!

Awesome, I responded. The bottom line is, as long as you love the results and you get the work done, I'm totally fine with you hating the work itself. High-five! See you next week.

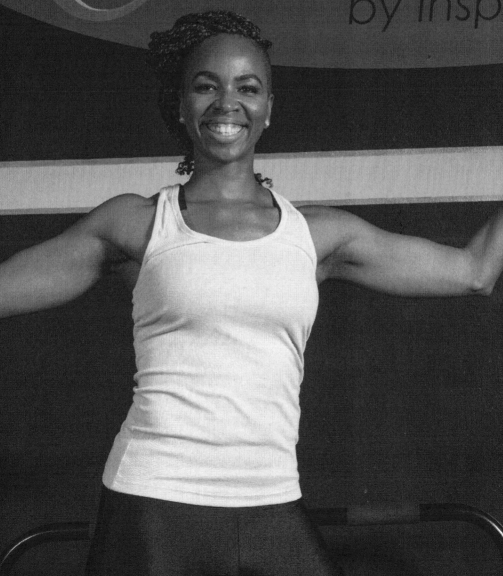

ABOUT YOUR COACH

It would take many years of nurturing before my love for self-care as a fitness professional and coach would blossom. My parents sparked my interest, but it was the physical challenges that I experienced as an adolescent that took my desires for improved self-care to greater heights. Like most teenagers I was inflexible and thought I knew everything. I was a loner, quietly driven and disciplined for someone my age. Later in life, that discipline and drive would both help and hurt me.

At age fourteen and a half, I developed cysts that would explode in my body, causing enough agony that anyone stricken with them would have fallen to their knees. I desperately wanted to get rid of them but my teenage brain never wanted to be a bother to anyone, especially my mom, so I decided to handle the situation on my own. Google wasn't around yet, so I learned what I could from my local library's encyclopedias, and used a phone book to complete my research. There was a nearby clinic that would confidentially treat teenagers like me. A soft shame settled in my gut. This would be my little secret.

The clinic was a strange and uncomfortable place. I had never gone to any doctor without my mother. The woman at the front desk was unfazed by my discomfort. She invited me through two sets of double doors into a fluorescent-lit room where she collected some of my basics; my height, weight, and blood pressure, etc. Once that was done, I was escorted to another room where I would be seen by the doctor.

I got the feeling that doctors at the clinic changed regularly. The doctor looked at my chart. Her silence made me nervous. There were no questions about my health or family history as I had anticipated; or even why I was there alone. I thought, "She thinks that I'm some orphan child without anyone to love and take care of them."

The doctor kept saying, "Hmmm." I wondered what she was thinking, but of course didn't ask, because you don't ask adults, especially doctors questions as a kid. Why was she making that noise? I thought. Her sounds created words that I finally understood. "I am scheduling you for minor surgery" My heart dropped. "Can I have surgery without my mother knowing about it?" She spoke again, "After the surgery, it is very likely that this will come right back, but at least it will temporarily relieve your pain." I was quiet. "Betty, my nurse will take your paperwork and add you to the schedule; I will see you in a few days."

I walked out of that clinic terrified. I needed a solution. I had no idea what I was getting myself into.

Surgery day came quickly. Here I was fourteen and a half and in way over my head.

Full of fear, I ushered myself to the clinic. Everything was happening so fast. Once I was in the back room with the doctor, I used my most confident voice to ask for an explanation of the surgical process. The doctor was unapologetically crude, "No, I don't think you need to know that. Let's just get started. " I took a deep breath.

The doctor pushed a needle into the area surrounding the cyst. I gasped a breath of death. She was anesthetizing me. I watched in terror as she used a small blade to slice my skin. With a damp gauze in hand, she applied intense pressure to the swollen area; a thick paste oozed. Heavy pressure was replaced then replaced by the discomfort of my skin being lifted and tugged. The doctor inserted a three-inch tube into the belly of the cyst. "I'm inserting this to allow for continual drainage." Silent tears fell from my eyes. She wiped the area clean and said. "Leave the tube in until your next visit; allow it to drain completely; and keep your hands and fingers away."

My teenage brain did not process all of her instructions. The horrible but predictable happened. I mistakenly let the wounded area come in contact with a liquid acid and when it did, I let out a screech so loud that I am sure my friends two streets over heard me. I frantically flooded the area with water. I thought the pain would never subside.

A tornado of feelings consumed me. I felt ashamed, sad and alone. Why was this happening to me? Frustrated and discouraged, I decided that I needed to get a handle on this. I was going to live pain-free for good. I took refuge in my mother's collection of books on cures for the body, detoxification, and healthy home remedies. I read all of them cover to cover. I decided that I needed a new way of living and being.

I put myself on a regimen. I ate a strict plant-based diet. I got up before dawn and exercised with television icons Denise Austin and Gilad Ganklowitz, whom I had been exercising with since I was ten years old. I used a massage technique around my cyst-prone area, something I had read about in my mom's reflexology book. I took herbal and salt infusion baths. I applied medicinal essential oils to my skin. I prayed, read and sung for and about my new pain free body. The changes I needed to make for healthy living were easy for me. I was in control of my body and that felt great.

The human experience is funny, though. Today, I can remember the horror of my first cyst, the painful surgery, and when I decided to change my lifestyle. But I can't remember the first time I felt no pain. I only remember that it wasn't instant and that several months after the surgery I asked myself, "Why didn't the doctor recommend a lifestyle change? Why was surgery the first and only option she offered?"

YOUR MANTRA

I choose to live, work, play and pray smart. I choose to improve. Everyday I live my life with and on purpose.

FITNESS TRAINING TIPS

Three weeks of consistent movement, you are amazing! Do remain steadfast on your journey and continue to work at a pace that feels good to you. Keep in mind, cardiovascular, strength, mobility and flexibility training are still your primary exercise objectives.

by Inspire Me Fit

FEEL IT!

Week Three

WORKOUT FOR DETOXIFICATION

by Inspire Me Fit

IT'S WARM-UP TIME, LET'S ROLL

- Hit this workout at least **four times this week**!

- Our goal is to clean house on our bodies and lives. We have been working on improving the way that we think, what we consume and now, how we feel. And, if you are like most people, you'll agree with me that it feels good to move in a way that makes us stronger, fitter, and better. So, keep going because **the best results are yet to come!**

- Do each movement for 30 – 60 seconds and repeat it two to three times before beginning your strength work. Take your time, make your moves as big as possible, and go at a slow to medium pace.

SUPINE ROLL UPS

- Be sure to sit tall to start

- Lead your roll down by pulling in your lower abs. Try to create the internal feeling of cutting off your urine flow. Repeat this on the way up

- Allow your low back to touch the floor first, then your middle and finally your upper back

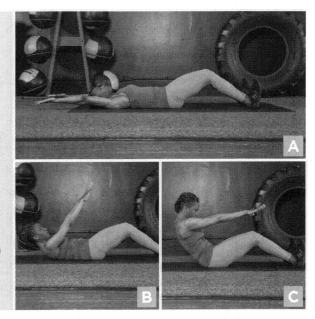

SUPINE SINGLE LEG CROSS OVER

- Fully extend your body

- Lift one leg as high as you can comfortably

- Keep your shoulders down while tapping your lifted leg towards the floor

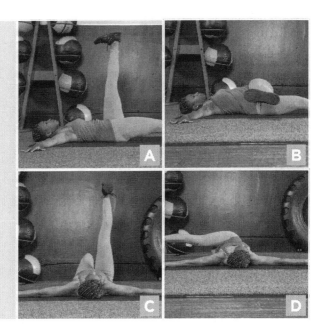

STANDING HIGH KNEES OR HIGH KNEE MARCH

- You have the option to jump or not with this exercise

- Make your movements as big as possible

- If you are jumping, be sure to land softly

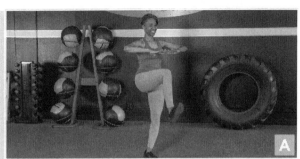

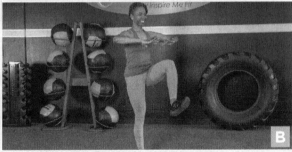

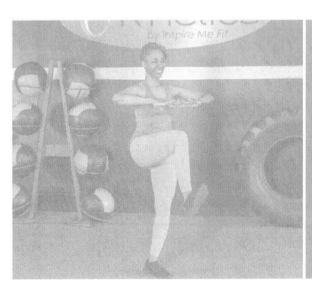

TIP OF THE DAY

Do your best to not let your mind float during your working out. **Be present!**

Focus on the muscles that you're working. The more focused you are, the more likely you will execute the exercise properly.

STRENGTH WORKOUT

COMPLETE EXERCISES AS FOLLOWS:

- 30 seconds of work for beginners with a maximum of 60 seconds of rest between exercises

- 60 seconds of work for intermediate to advanced exercisers with a maximum of 30 seconds of rest between exercises

- 60 seconds of work for advanced exercisers with no rest between exercises

- Go in this order: leg, push, hinge and pull exercises; Complete two to four sets

- Complete one to two sets of cool-down exercises once your strength work is done

LEG EXERCISES

WIDE STANCE SQUAT

- Begin with your legs wide

- Your toes should be turned out to two o'clock and ten o'clock

- Keep your knees, ankles and feet in the same alignment

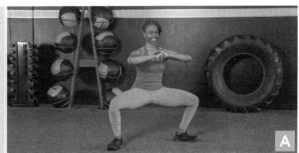
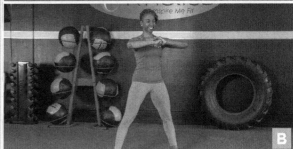

GOOD MORNINGS

- Stand as tall as you can

- Pull your elbows back as much as you can with your arms behind your head

- Hinge forward, aiming for a flat back

- Soften your knees, but don't lock them

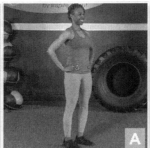
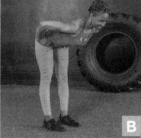
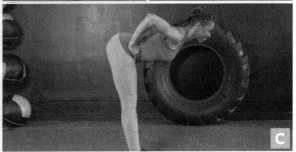

REAR LUNGE TO HIGH KNEE

- Start in a lunge position

- Raise your knee, pulling it into the belly as tightly as you can

- Stand tall on your supporting leg

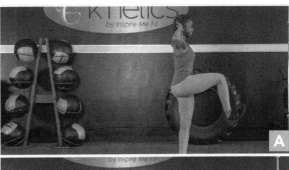
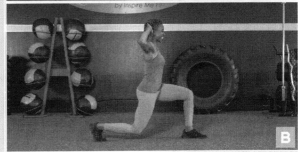

PUSHES EXERCISES

PUSH UP WITH LATERAL ARM EXTENSION

- Assume your push-up position

- When coming up, extend one arm out to the side

- Be sure the keep your hips as level as possible

- Make the exercise easier by dropping your knees to the floor

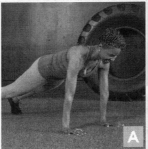
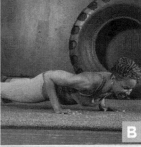
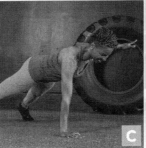
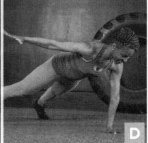

FREE WEIGHT SKULL CRUSHER

- Lie on a sturdy flat surface

- Bend your elbows towards the ceiling

- Extend your arms fully, holding your free weight

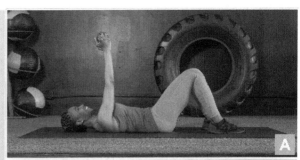

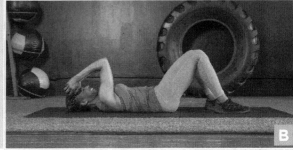

"A" FRAME CHEST PRESS

- Lie on a sturdy surface

- Bring your weights towards your chest in the shape of the letter "A"

- Press your weights up towards the ceiling into a horizontal position

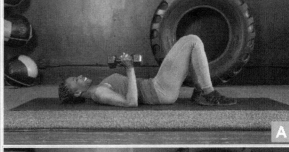

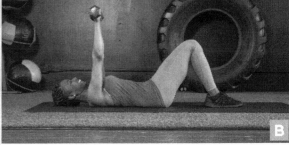

HINGE EXERCISES

RISING BOAT

- Start by lying flat on your back

- Bring your body up in one piece

- Raise your feet away from the floor, or keep your toes planted

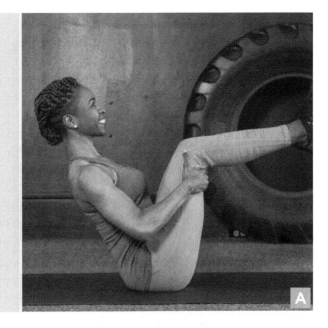

FOREARM PLANK HOLD

- Come into a low plank position

- Engage your abs to support your low back

- Take a wide stance to make the plank a little easier and a narrow one to make the plank more challenging

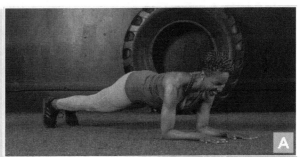

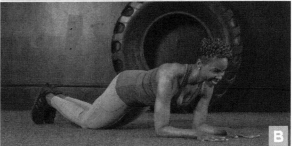

SUPINE FLUTTER KICKS

- Lie flat on your back

- Engage your low abs while lifting your legs to a position that feels challenging but not overwhelming

- Make small kicks with your legs

- Bend your knees slightly if you cannot lift your legs comfortably

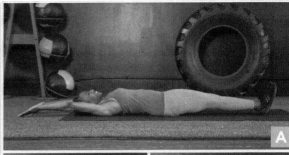
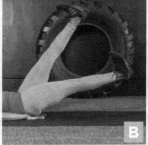
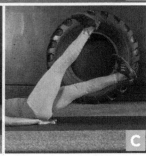

PULLS EXERCISES

FREE WEIGHT LAT PULL DOWN

- Take a wall sit

- Holding a light set of weights, lift and lower your arms

- Be sure that your low back pushes firmly against the wall

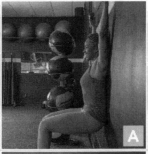
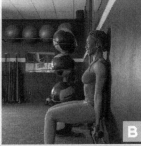
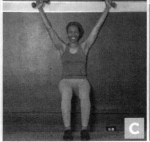
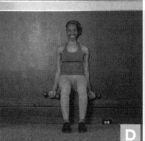

PRONE WEIGHTED SUPER HERO

- Start with your belly resting on the floor

- Extend your arms into the letter "V"

- Pull your arms down by your sides and then back to "V" position

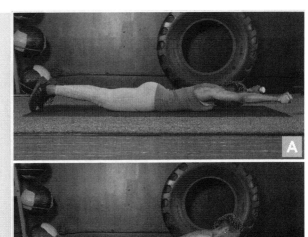

STANDING REVERSE FLY

- From a standing position, bring your chest parallel to the floor

- Maintain a flat back

- Slightly bend your elbows

- Raise your arms back and behind yourself with the goal of pinching the shoulder blades back and behind yourself

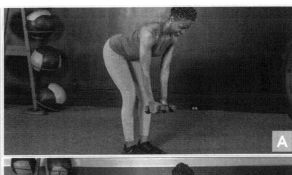

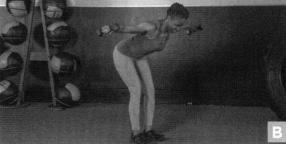

COOL-DOWN STRETCHES

HAMSTRING STRETCH

- Place one leg on a sturdy surface

- Stand tall

- Extend your torso towards your raised leg

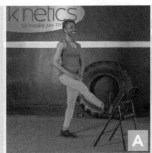
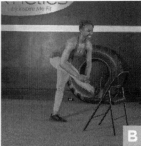
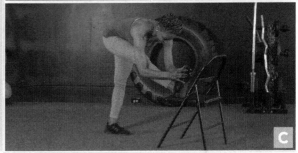

SIDE LUNGE STRETCH

- Stand tall with your legs in a straddle

- Be sure your feet are turned out

- Bend one knee with the goal of stretching your straight leg

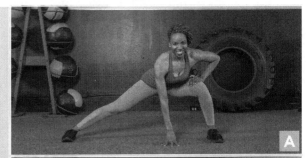
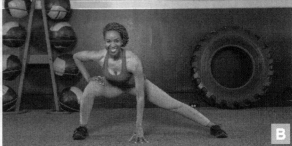

STRADDLED FORWARD BEND

- Start by standing tall

- Place your arms high in the air

- Hinge from the hips, extending your spine as long as you can

- Fold forward to bend

- Interlock your elbows to dangle forward

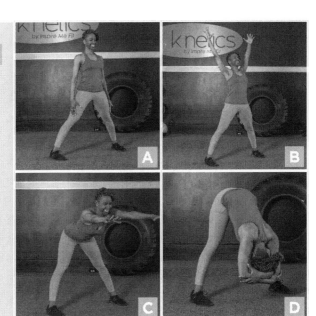

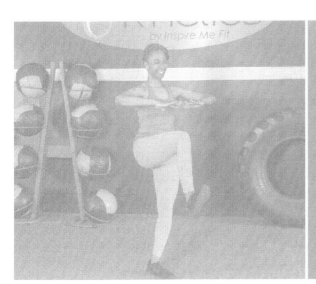

TIP OF THE DAY

If you are just beginning a workout regimen or you're ramping things up, It will likely take you thirty days of consistent work to see changes in your body.

Don't self-sabotage by stopping or stalling before you reach that point.

LIVE LIFE TOOL

Music! Allow this playlist to motivate you.

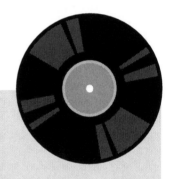

FEEL IT! MOTIVATIONAL PLAYLIST

- **I Feel Good** by James Brown
- **Are You Gonna Go My Way** by Lenny Kravitz
- **Keep Your Head Up** by Andy Grammar
- **Can't Stop the Feeling** by Justin Timberlake
- **Happy** by Pharrell
- **Victorious** by Wolfmother
- **Feel Invincible** by Skillet
- **Work** by Lil John
- **Head Above Water** by Avril Lavigne
- **Sabotage** by the Beastie Boys

7 DAY READ IT AND EAT IT SAMPLE MENU FOR DETOXIFICATION

DAY 1

Pre-breakfast: 8 ounce glass of lemon or lime water, either warm or room temperature

Breakfast: green drink of your choice, and your choice of either decaf coffee or tea

Lunch: vegetarian bento box with your choice of side salad

Dinner: carrot ginger soup with a side salad

Snack options: This week choose one piece (or 1/2 cup) of fresh fruit, sliced raw vegetables (avoid sweet vegetables like carrots or beets this week) and/or one serving of any non-sweet snack found in the snack recipes section. To achieve the best fat loss results, limit snack foods to 300 calories for less. Do your best to consume 64-80 ounces of water today while keeping your sodium intake to 2,000mg total or less.

DAY 2

Pre-breakfast: 8 ounce glass of lemon or lime water, either warm or room temperature

Breakfast: protein drink of choice with either your choice of decaf coffee or tea

Lunch: Asian Vegetable Stir Fry, steamed cauliflower rice and your choice side salad

Dinner: cream of spinach soup with your choice side salad

Snack options: This week choose one piece (or 1/2 cup) of fresh fruit, sliced raw vegetables (avoid sweet vegetables like carrots or beets this week) and/or one serving of any non-sweet snack found in the snack recipes section. To achieve the best fat loss results, limit snack foods to 300 calories for less. Do your best to consume 64-80 ounces of water today while keeping your sodium intake to 2,000mg total or less.

DAY 3

Pre-breakfast: 8 ounce glass of lemon or lime water, either warm or room temperature

Breakfast: quarter of a cup cream of quinoa, fresh fruit and your choice of either decaf coffee or tea

Lunch: vegetarian or pescatarian bento box with your choice of side salad

Dinner: Queen B black-eyed peas and steamed cauliflower rice

Snack options: This week choose one piece (or 1/2 cup) of fresh fruit, sliced raw vegetables (avoid sweet vegetables like carrots or beets this week) and/or one serving of any non-sweet snack found in the snack recipes section. To achieve the best fat loss results, limit snack foods to 300 calories for less. Do your best to consume 64-80 ounces of water today while keeping your sodium intake to 2,000mg total or less.

DAY 4

Pre-breakfast: 8 ounce glass of lemon or lime water, either warm or room temperature

Breakfast: omelet of your choice with your choice of decaf coffee or tea

Lunch: grilled fish or seitan, mixed greens, and one serving of your choice of beans or peas

Dinner: vegetable broth and your choice of side salad

Snack options: This week choose one piece (or 1/2 cup) of fresh fruit, sliced raw vegetables (avoid sweet vegetables like carrots or beets this week) and/or one serving of any non-sweet snack found in the snack recipes section. To achieve the best fat loss results, limit snack foods to 300 calories for less. Do your best to consume 64-80 ounces of water today while keeping your sodium intake to 2,000mg total or less.

DAY 5

Pre-breakfast: 8 ounce glass of lemon or lime water, either warm or room temperature

Breakfast: green drink of your choice with your choice of decaf coffee or tea

Lunch: vegetarian steak, mixed greens and one serving of raw nuts and/or seeds

Dinner: black bean soup with your choice of side salad

Snack options: This week choose one piece (or 1/2 cup) of fresh fruit, sliced raw vegetables (avoid sweet vegetables like carrots or beets this week) and/or one serving of any non-sweet snack found in the snack recipes section. To achieve the best fat loss results, limit snack foods to 300 calories for less. Do your best to consume 64-80 ounces of water today while keeping your sodium intake to 2,000 mg total or less.

DAY 6

Pre-breakfast: 8 ounce glass of lemon or lime water, either warm or room temperature

Breakfast: protein drink of your choice with your choice of either decaf coffee or tea

Lunch: zoodle mac & cheese with your choice of side salad

Dinner: vegetable broth with large salad

Snack options: This week choose one piece (or 1/2 cup) of fresh fruit, sliced raw vegetables (avoid sweet vegetables like carrots or beets this week) and/or one serving of any non-sweet snack found in the snack recipes section. To achieve the best fat loss results, limit snack foods to 300 calories for less. Do your best to consume 64-80 ounces of water today while keeping your sodium intake to 2,000 mg total or less.

DAY 7

Pre-breakfast: 8 ounce glass of lemon or lime water, either warm or room temperature

Breakfast: omelet of your choice with either decaf coffee or tea

Lunch: cauliflower meatballs & gravy with your choice of side salad

Dinner: hearty vegetable soup with your choice of side salad

Snack options: This week choose one piece (or 1/2 cup) of fresh fruit, sliced raw vegetables (avoid sweet vegetables like carrots or beets this week) and/or one serving of any non-sweet snack found in the snack recipes section. To achieve the best fat loss results, limit snack foods to 300 calories for less. Do your best to consume 64-80 ounces of water today while keeping your sodium intake to 2,000 mg total or less.

Wow, you made it to week four and it wasn't so bad, right? This week we'll look at how we can live a detox life to the fullest. We'll learn how to enjoy the progress we've made, and take it to the next level over and over again.

Pick your favorite quote and post it where it can be seen often!

LIVE IT!

CALL TO ACTION

The going got tough but I got tougher

"How to win in Life:
1. work hard,
2. complain less,
3. listen more,
4. try, learn, and grow,
5. don't let people tell you it can't be done,
6. make no excuses."

GERMANY KENT

Her heart was beating fast. She could hardly think. She looked to her right and caught a glimpse of a small-framed golden-brown woman vigorously stretching. To her left was a mature man dancing non-stop like Mohammed Ali. There were thousands of people at race day. She couldn't believe that after twelve months, she was actually living her dream to run the New York City Marathon. This would be one of the best days of her life. The loudspeaker sounded, "Runners are you ready?" The runners roared YES! The race gun popped, and as she took off with all the runners, an electric surge ran through Lina's feet. Her eyes watered with joy. "How in the world did I get here?" she thought.

In her training group, Lina's assignment had been to select images from a magazine that would capture her short and long-term goals. Her collage was simple. It had four magazine clippings. The one dead center read: qualify and run the New York City Marathon. My commitments are to:

1. Take care of my body in every way that I can

2. Meet the requirements for the race

3. Work on my ability to run five days per week

Lina was excited, nervous, and committed all at once. She got to work immediately.

Twelve hard months of training felt like forever, especially on cold rainy days. But Lina had made a decision, and she wasn't going to give up just because a little challenge was knocking at her door. She decided to plunge forward, running in the heat, rain, snow, and cold. Lina ran on good days and bad. She ran with friends or alone. Lina ran because the goal that she had set for herself was important. She ran because she knew that if she could make this happen, she could make anything happen.

Receiving her qualifying email was surreal. Sure, she had run the required number of short and long races needed to apply for the New York City Marathon, but being selected out of the thousands of people who'd applied, well, that made her feel downright special, like this was a dream come true. Her heart and eyes filled with joy. She kept working towards her goals, waiting for race day to finally show its gorgeous face.

The run itself was both bitter and sweet. The terrain was tough at times. Sweat poured from her brow as she focused on lifting one leg after the other, each one feeling like a ton of bricks. Running through the city boroughs, that was something different. That was beautiful. Hundreds smiled and clapped in support. Lina's heart filled with joy. Mile twenty was the toughest. She felt as if her entire body was shutting down. Her mind took over. "This is just a small moment in time. Lina, pass the next tree. Good, now the next stop sign, awesome, now the next person." Everything is possible with a lot of commitment and continuous effort. She kept deliberate, positive self talk for five life-changing miles. Then, mile twenty-five showed its empathetic face and Lina wept. "This was hard but I would do it all again. I am so grateful."

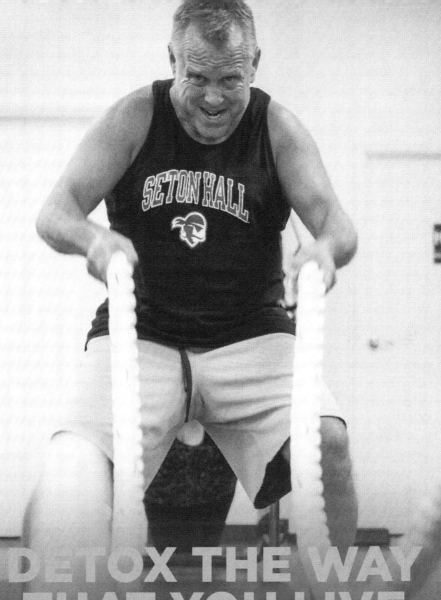

DETOX THE WAY THAT YOU LIVE

YOUR COACH'S ADVICE:

Personal greatness is not optional, it's our human duty! Expect that it will require hard work. Get it done, see your trend of awesomeness and celebrate yourself for making it happen!

It's all about having a plan

"By failing to prepare, you are preparing to fail."

BENJAMIN FRANKLIN

The environment was toxic. He wasn't sure how he would reconcile what was happening, but he knew it had to be done. The thought of the separation was eating away at him, but the pain of pretending like everything was okay felt like a wound that he was sure wouldn't stop bleeding on its own. He had done all that he could but still, it wasn't enough. Word had come down the pipeline that he would be fired at the end of the month and there was nothing that he could do. His job was done.

Pete was sliding into a depression. He would no longer be the primary breadwinner in his family. He felt weak and inadequate, and he was clear that it would not be long before he would feel overwhelmed and turn again to the one thing that had always brought him relief, food. Pete's eyes filled with tears. He was terrified. His wife would leave him, and his children would hate him. They had gone through so much the last time that he was severely depressed. It was bad; he was homebound, miserable and one-hundred-and-seven pounds heavier. He was clear that if he backslid, his fear and lack of self-confidence had put his family through hell. He was not willing to do that again.

With his back towards his office door, Pete sat low in his chair. He tried to hear his therapist's words in his head. He thought about the hundreds of hours that he had spent journaling. What was he going to do? Pete thought, "How did I survive that?" He was alone but blurted out his response. "I need help. I need to give my therapist a call," and before he could talk himself out of it, Pete picked up the phone and began dialing.

Cheryl had been his saving grace in the past, and this time was no different. She answered his call on the very first ring. "Peter, it's been a long time. How are you?" "Not great, can I come in to see you? I can feel myself sliding down a rocky road and I'm not sure what to do." Cheryl met with Peter that same day. She reminded him of what they had worked through before.

"Pete, you have taken the very first and most important step in managing your symptoms of depression, and that is recognizing that you need help. Thank you for that. The next thing that we have to do is call your wife. Secrets of this magnitude are never a good thing. Your wife is a loving woman; she will help you work through this. Let's give her a call now." Peter dialed Tina and reluctantly told her everything. It wasn't long before the three of them had devised a resilience plan. The key for Peter was that he had a plan. He'd find a professional to help him update his resume. He'd contact a corporate headhunter to start working on other opportunities. As a family, they would tighten their financial belts and avoid senseless spending. And Peter would call his old personal fitness trainer and dive into a sixty-day fitness challenge. His trainer would create structure and accountability, and the fitness challenge would create healthy competition while allowing him to encourage his teammates. Peter had a plan, support, and newfound hope. He was ready to take action.

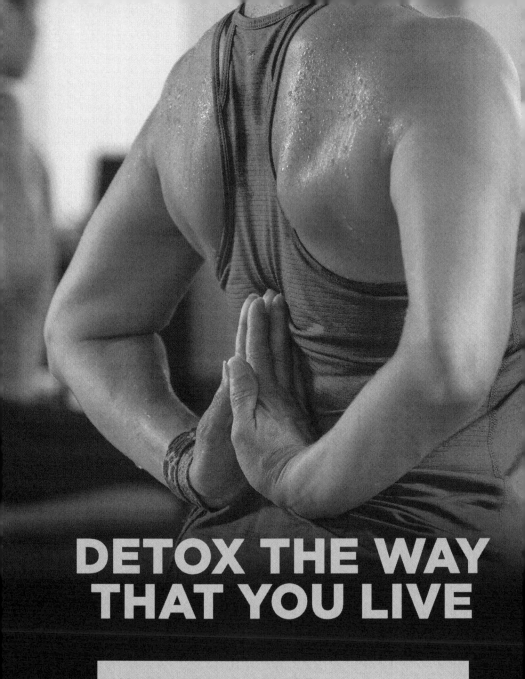

DETOX THE WAY THAT YOU LIVE

YOUR COACH'S ADVICE:

When you ask to be something other than who you are, the outcome may not be what you want it to be. So, it is best to work towards being the best version of your authentic self.

I want more

For the longest time I just didn't see the point of putting all that extra stress on my body. My life has always been full of activity. I love gardening. I shovel snow like a champion. Every three-thousand miles I lift the hood of my Ford and give it the oil change that it needs. I figured, if I could do all of that, I don't really need to know how to do a push-up, do I? Joan was right. If her only goal was to only be active, maybe her current lifestyle would have been enough to sustain her. But, that wasn't her only goal. She wanted more physical strength, upper arm definition – particularly in what she called her saggy back-arm, as well as a lifted bottom and removal of the slowly forming pouch around her belly button. She loved her body but she did not like the recent changes that she saw it making. "Honestly," she said during her transformation consultation, "My body is being downright disrespectful. I feel as if I am giving it very specific instructions but after twelve months of deliberate extra activity nothing has improved. My mood is low and I'm angry."

"Joan, I get your frustration and there are definitely ways to turn this around. You are a healthy, an able bodied person. We just need to take a slightly different approach." "I'm listening," she said. "What are some of your favorite activities?" "I enjoy hiking, reading, writing and hanging out with friends." "That's wonderful. Let's build a detox regimen that allows you to do all of those things plus a few others that aren't your favorite but that you are willing to do such as a higher intensity interval style training with a trainer. Let's also, shift your diet to include a nutrient dense plant-based regimen that is low in starch and fruit but and high in healthy fats. Additionally, I would like for you to monitor your urine making sure that it is always pale yellow to clear as well as your bowel movements." "Why my bowel movements," she grunted. "Waste of any sorts sitting inside of you for too long is bound to have a negative effect so let's help your body excrete waste regularly. I'd also like for you to watch this documentary on how to be happy."

"I believe that you'll appreciate the stories presented and naturally shift into a happier way of being. Finally, do drown yourself in positive music. I am confident after thirty days of diligent work; we will be in a much better place." They smiled and Joan got to work.

KAY'S SUCCESS STORY

Pushing Past Fear

*"You gain strength, courage, and confidence by every
experience in which you really stop to look fear in the
face. You are able to say to yourself, 'I lived through this
horror. I can take the next thing that comes along."*

ELEANOR ROOSEVELT

K ay turned over in her bed. She had only slept three hours that night. She glanced at the clock, 8:59AM, uggh! It was already time to wake up. She had thirty minutes to collect herself, shower and head to the pool. Today was her very first swim meet. She reluctantly moved around the house, thinking that all of those grueling days of waking up at 4:00AM to practice had to have made a difference. She heard her coach's encouraging voice in her head. "Four laps, breaststroke; Kay, you can beat this time, and I know you can." At those practices. Kay had screamed on the inside, "My arms feel like jello, my fingers like raisins, and I'm starving. I hate my mother for making me do this." But she'd reached the wall, flipped and powered forward with great speed and force. Today was a big deal. Today she'd be a lead swimmer and she couldn't let her team down.

She arrived just in time to meet her teammates. They seemed so calm. She thought, "I am not good enough to be here. I could get out of this if I mysteriously got sick. Yep, I feel sick in a way." Kay convinced herself that Jordan would lead swim and that the team would win and they'd all celebrate. Just as she was having that thought, her coach Ronnie tapped her on the shoulder. "I know that you're afraid but you don't have to be. You are ready. Let go of all those negative thoughts of fear, self doubt, and lack, and push forward like the lion I know that you are. All the power that you will ever need is inside of you. Fear not." Oh, man, Kay thought, what was coach doing inside of her head? Kay breathed a forceful sigh. "I guess I don't have a choice. I'll go change."

Kay felt as if the warm-up was happening in slow motion. One by one, each swimmer gracefully plunged into the cold water. Kay went deep inside of herself. Her toned arms lifted as she dove into the water. She warmed up with twelve laps of her freestyle stroke. She flipped onto her back and allowed the mermaid flap of her feet to create a momentum that would help her glide past three of her swim mates. She flipped again; this was it, the stroke that her arms were made for, breaststroke. Kay lifted, flew up for a gulp of breath and back down into the water. She felt good. Kay looked up to see her coach's smiling face. She decided then and there that she would win. Success was the only option at this point. Kay leaped out of the water, threw on her towel and her headset. She was ready.

The soft chatter of her team surrounded her. She felt their love and support but she would need to stay tapped into her greater self in order to make winning a reality. The digital clock above her read 12:01PM. She was next up. Kay closed her eyes, removed her towel and headset, and headed for her lane. She repeated, I am Kay, I am a winner. The "go" alarm sounded, and she went. Kay repeated to herself, I am a winner. I was born to win. The competition pulled ahead. Not today, she thought. They were now moving in sync with each other. To win, Kay would have to have a lot of power behind her next flip. She touched the underwater wall first. She was in the lead. All she had to do is stay focused, and her body would naturally do the rest.

- Lift, breathe, pull, she commanded internally.

- Lift, breathe, and pull

- Lift, breathe, and pull

She touched the wall and could hear a roaring crowd. Was it true; had she won? Kay held the pool wall and turned towards the clock. She'd swum her best time ever. She couldn't believe it. Kay started crying. She met her coach's eyes and they both said, Thank you!

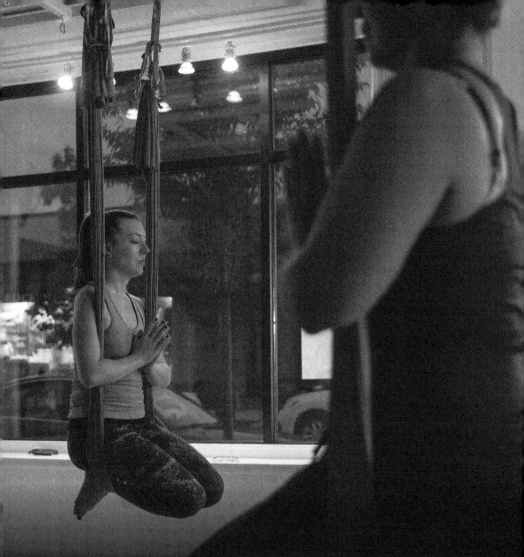

DETOX THE WAY THAT YOU LIVE

YOUR COACH'S ADVICE:

Shift your thoughts on failure. It is not a bad thing. It fact I believe it is a powerful opportunity to learn from your life.

LIVE LIFE TOOL

It is unfortunate but in most cases true; what we see we believe. Do yourself a favor and watch things that create positive and powerful emotions; this will create the platform needed for your future positive and powerful actions . See a list of powerful and uplifting movies on Appendix page 186.

ABOUT YOUR COACH

There was a fire brewing in me. I was both excited and afraid. It had worked. I'd convinced my boss that we should take twenty students on an adventure 4,990 miles away. My stomach sank with happy terror. I had no contacts there, and knew only what I'd read in books. It didn't matter though; my career was on the line. This was my idea and I needed to figure it out! We were going to West Africa on a cultural dance adventure.

On the day of my departure I was jittery. Everything was riding on this. My husband dropped me off at the airport with plenty of time to spare. I checked my bags and waited. I waited so long in the wrong area that I missed my flight. Anxiousness got the best of me. I panicked. Everything was riding on this.

It took ten for me to calm down and collected myself. This would not end my career. "I'm in charge. Woman up, Metra," I said to myself. I dove into solutions mode. Rearrange your schedule. Call your husband. Stay put for tonight and fly out tomorrow. You are not about to punk out I thought to myself. I put my big girl panties on, got to my destination and had one of the best experiences of my life!

Life just wouldn't be life if the terrain was all flat. Nope, living means that there will always be mountains to climb. The key to climbing those mountains is perseverance.

YOUR MANTRA

Giving up on me isn't even an option. Today and everyday I forgive myself for not being perfect. I give myself permission to make mistakes and bounce back with a greater sense of love and affection for who I am today as well as who I will become.

LIVE LIFE TOOL

Music! Use this playlist to boost your energy

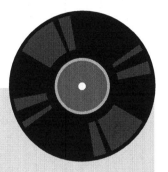

- **Living My Life Like It's Golden** by Jill Scott
- **The Whistle Song** by Frankie Knuckles
- **Roar** by Katy Perry
- **Beat It** by Michael Jackson
- **Hiatus** by Defeat-EP
- **Light 'Em Up** Fall Out Boy Lyrics
- **The Script** by Hall of Fame ft. will.i.am
- **Level Up** by Ciara
- **Let's Move Your Body** by Beyonce
- **Barracuda** by Heart

LIVE LIFE WORKOUT

Life is for living. I encourage you to work hard and live hard. Living feels good when you feel healthy. Hit this workout at least four times this week. This week during your workout, concentrate on how amazing it feels to make positive change. Our goal is to create the very best version of you in terms of the way that you think, what you consume, how you feel, and how you live. We all only get one opportunity to make our lives amazing. Let's get to work at it.

LIVE IT!

Week Four

WORKOUT FOR DETOXIFICATION

IT'S WARM-UP TIME, LET'S GET TO IT!

- Do each movement for 30 – 60 seconds and repeat it two to three times before beginning your strength work.

- Take your time, make your moves as big as possible, and go at a slow to medium pace.

FORWARD SNAP KICK

- Do this in place or moving across the floor

- Stand tall as you kick

- Bend the knee, then extend the leg outward, pushing the heel out

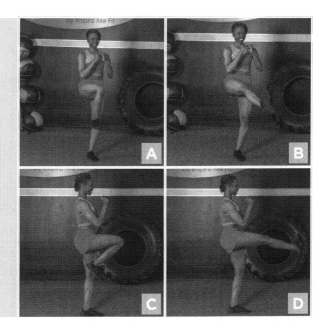

SIDE SNAP KICK

- From a standing position, shift your body weight onto one leg

- Kick outward, extending your leg fully

- Alternate sides

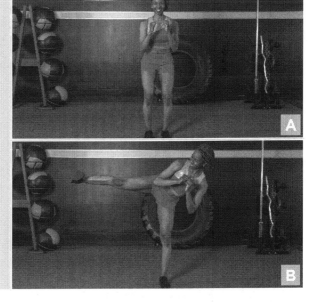

STANDING DONKEY KICK

- From a standing position, shift your body weight onto one leg

- Looking over your back shoulder, kick backwards

- If you can't maintain your balance, hold onto a sturdy surface

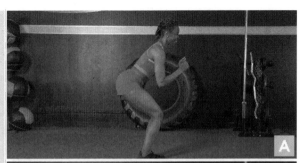
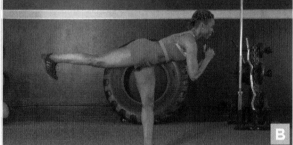

PLANK JACK

- From a high plank position, jump or step the legs wide and then together

- Keep your movements going at a rhythm that feels comfortable to you

- Engage your abs to avoid a lot of wiggling in your middle body

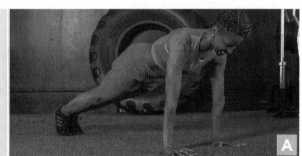
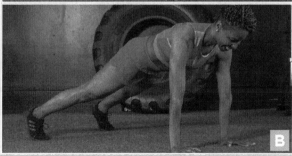

YOU ARE SO COMMITTED, KEEP UP THE GOOD WORK!

STRENGTH WORKOUT

COMPLETE EXERCISES AS FOLLOWS:

- 30 seconds of work for beginners with a maximum of 60 seconds of rest between exercises

- 60 seconds of work for intermediate to advanced exercisers with a maximum of 30 seconds of rest between exercises

- 60 seconds of work for advanced exercisers with no rest between exercises

- Go in this order: legs, push, hinge and pull exercises; Complete two to four sets

- Complete one to two sets of cool-down exercises once your strength work is done

LEG EXERCISES

VICTORY SQUATS

- Stand tall, with your feet slightly wider than hip distance apart

- Turn your feet outward to a comfortable position

- Fully extend your arms into a "V"

- Maintain a lifted chest the entire time

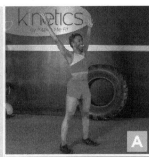 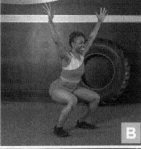
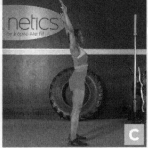 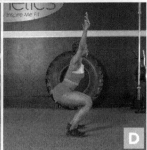

WALL SIT LEG LIFT

- Lean against the wall for your wall sit and extend one leg

- Position your other leg towards the midline of your body

- With your hands against the wall, raise your extended leg away from the floor as high as you can without taking your low back off the wall

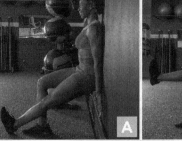 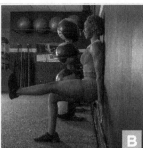
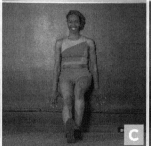 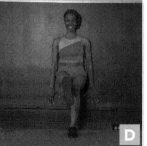

KNEELING LUNGE TO STAND

- Start in a single-leg kneeling position

- Stand tall, moving through a lunge into straight legs

- If keeping your balance is an issue, hold onto a sturdy surface for support. Work toward getting rid of the support

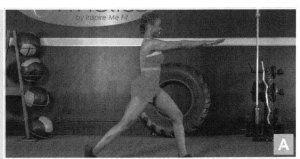

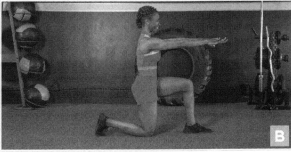

PUSH EXERCISES

NARROW TO WIDE PUSH-UP

- Bring your body into a wide-armed push-up position

- Hit a single push-up

- Then pull your hands closer together, creating a heart shape

- Hit another single push-up

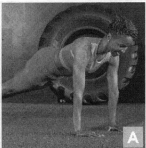
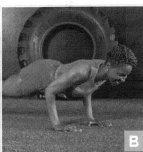
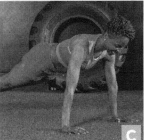
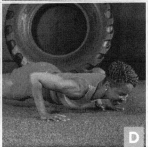

TRICEP KICK BACK

- Use a medium to light weight

- Hinge forward from your hips, bringing your chest towards parallel to the floor

- Bring the weights to your shoulders, bending your elbows, then behind your back with your arms fully extended

- Don't move your wrists

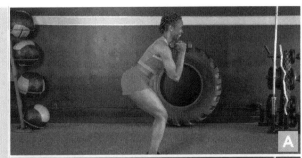
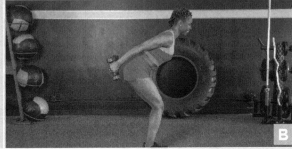

HALF SQUAT TO SHOULDER PRESS

- From a squat position, rest your weights on your shoulders

- Sit as low as you can, then come into a full standing position

- Press the weights up high and rotate them to a horizontal position

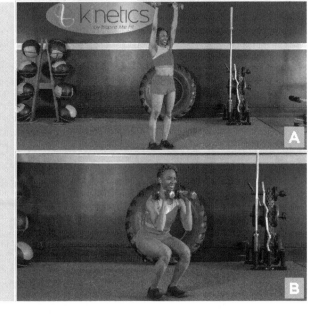

HINGE EXERCISES

SUPINE DOUBLE LEG CIRCLES

- Lie flat on your back
- Plaster your low back to the floor
- Bend both knees, bringing them into your chest
- Extend your legs upward towards the ceiling, then lower them towards the floor
- Only go as low as you can, keeping your back on the floor
- Reverse your circular direction

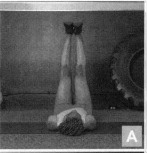
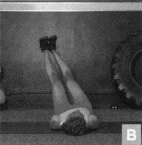
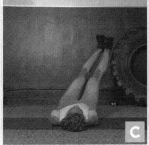
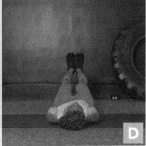

INCH WORM

- Start in a full plank position
- Walk your feet as far forward as you can
- Walk your feet back to plank
- Engage your abs to maintain a flat back

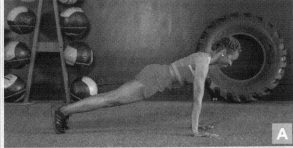
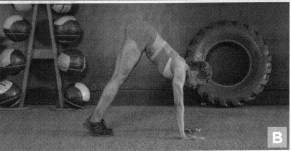

SUPINE DOUBLE LEG "I"

- Lie flat on your back
- Start by bending your knees into your chest
- Extend your legs upward, then open and close them to form the top of the letter "I"
- Once your legs are together again, lower them towards the floor so that it feels challenging in your abdomen but your low back is still on the floor
- Once at the lowest point, open and close your legs again, creating the bottom shape of the letter "I"

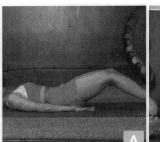
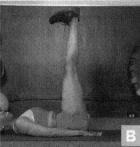
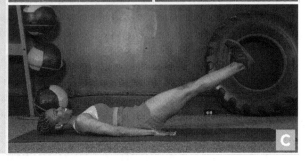

PULL EXERCISES

SEATED RESISTANCE BAND ROW

- Wrap your resistance band around the base of your feet
- Make sure that your feet are slightly wider than hip-width apart
- Criss-cross the bands and pull them tight until your arms are in line with your waist on either side

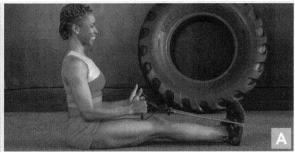
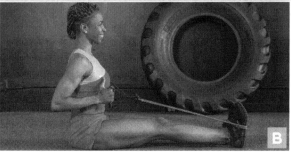

STANDING UPRIGHT ROW

- Step on your resistance bands

- Hold the bands so that your thumbs are facing inward

- Pull the bands upward towards your chin, creating the letter "v" with your elbows

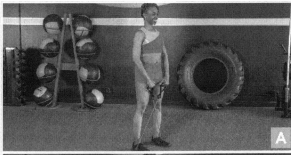

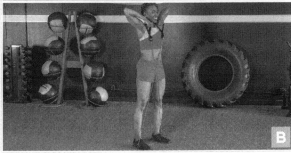

OVERHEAD EXTENSION WITH "T" PULL

- Begin in a standing position

- Bring the resistance band over your head into the letter "V"

- Pull the band tightly back until you create the letter "T"

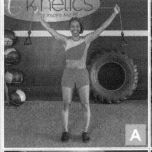
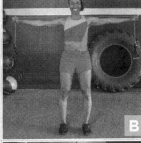
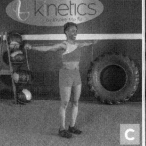
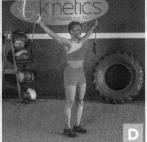

COOL-DOWN STRETCHES

HAPPY MORNING STRETCH

- Start in a seated position

- Sweep your legs to one side

- Place one hand on the floor

- Lift your body and your opposite hand in the direction of your bent knees

- Alternate sides

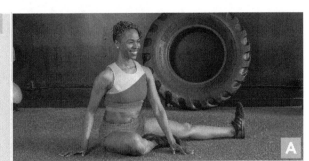
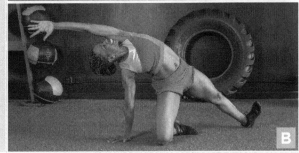

MODIFIED YOGA PIGEON STRETCH

- From a seated position, sweep your legs to one side

- Look at the leg that is in front and try align your shin with the wall in front of you

- Walk your hands wide and bring your upper body over your front leg

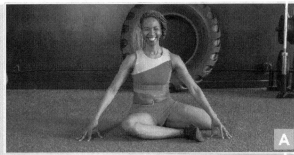
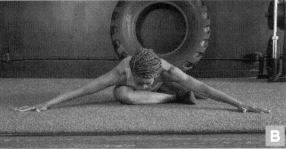

SEATED BUTTERFLY STRETCH

- From a seated position, bend your knees and bring the soles of your feet together

- Push your feet open as if you are reading a book

- Place your elbows down onto your knees

- Push your knees down towards the floor

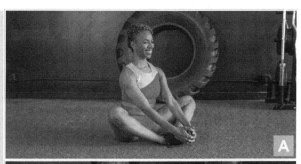

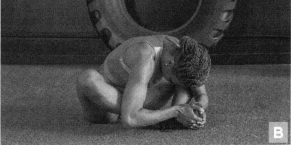

I AM TOTALLY CLAPPING FOR YOU! YOU DID A FANTASTIC JOB!

7 DAY READ IT AND EAT IT SAMPLE MENU FOR DETOXIFICATION

DAY 1

Pre-breakfast: 8 ounce glass of lemon or lime water, either warm or room temperature

Breakfast: smoothie of your choice with your choice of either decaf coffee or tea

Lunch: open-face black bean burger with your choice of a side salad

Dinner: your choice of soup with a side salad

Snack options: This week choose one piece (or 1/2 cup) of fresh fruit, sliced raw vegetables (avoid sweet vegetables like carrots or beets this week) and/or one serving of any non-sweet snack found in the snack recipes section. To achieve the best fat loss results, limit snack foods to 300 calories for less. Do your best to consume 64-80 ounces of water today while keeping your sodium intake to 2,000mg total or less.

DAY 2

Pre-breakfast: 8 ounce glass of lemon or lime water, either warm or room temperature e

Breakfast: protein drink of your choice with either decaf coffee or tea

Lunch: vegan or pescatarian bento box with your choice of a side salad

Dinner: hearty vegetable soup and your choice of a side salad

Snack options: This week choose one piece (or 1/2 cup) of fresh fruit, sliced raw vegetables (avoid sweet vegetables like carrots or beets this week) and/or one serving of any non-sweet snack found in the snack recipes section. To achieve the best fat loss results, limit snack foods to 300 calories for less. Do your best to consume 64-80 ounces of water today while keeping your sodium intake to 2,000 mg total or less.

DAY 3

Pre-breakfast: 8 ounce glass of lemon or lime water, either warm or room temperature

Breakfast: green drink of your choice with your choice of either decaf coffee or tea

Lunch: steamed vegetables and spices over cauliflower rice

Dinner: sweet potato crumb soup with your choice of side salad

Snack options: This week choose one piece (or 1/2 cup) of fresh fruit, sliced raw vegetables (avoid sweet vegetables like carrots or beets this week) and/or one serving of any non-sweet snack found in the snack recipes section. To achieve the best fat loss results, limit snack foods to 300 calories for less. Do your best to consume 64-80 ounces of water today while keeping your sodium intake to 2,000mg total or less.

DAY 4

Pre-breakfast: 8 ounce glass of lemon or lime water, either warm or room temperature

Breakfast: cup of coconut or soy yogurt with your choice of either decaf coffee or tea

Lunch: sautéed lentils and onions over steamed cauliflower rice with your choice of side salad

Dinner: Jenny's split pea soup and your choice of side salad

Snack options: This week choose one piece (or 1/2 cup) of fresh fruit, sliced raw vegetables (avoid sweet vegetables like carrots or beets this week) and/or one serving of any non-sweet snack found in the snack recipes section. To achieve the best fat loss results, limit snack foods to

300 calories for less. Do your best to consume 64-80 ounces of water today while keeping your sodium intake to 2,000mg total or less.

DAY 5

Pre-breakfast: 8 ounce glass of lemon or lime water, either warm or room temperature

Breakfast: smoothie of your choice with either decaf coffee or tea

Lunch: Healthy Happy Nachos with your choice of side salad

Dinner: vegetable broth with your choice of side salad

Snack options: This week choose one piece (or 1/2 cup) of fresh fruit, sliced raw vegetables (avoid sweet vegetables like carrots or beets this week) and/or one serving of any non-sweet snack found in the snack recipes section. To achieve the best fat loss results, limit snack foods to 300 calories for less. Do your best to consume 64-80 ounces of water today while keeping your sodium intake to 2,000mg total or less.

DAY 6

Pre-breakfast: 8 ounce glass of lemon or lime water, either warm or room temperature

Breakfast: green drink of your choice with your choice of either decaf coffee or tea

Lunch: vegetarian stuffed cabbage with your choice of side salad

Dinner: cream of spinach soup with your choice of side salad

Snack options: This week choose one piece (or 1/2 cup) of fresh fruit, sliced raw vegetables (avoid sweet vegetables like carrots or beets this week) and/or one serving of any non-sweet snack found in the snack recipes section. To achieve the best fat loss results, limit snack foods to 300 calories for less. Do your best to consume 64-80 ounces of water today while keeping your sodium intake to 2,000mg total or less.

DAY 7

Pre-breakfast: 8 ounce glass of lemon or lime water, either warm or room temperature

Breakfast: smoothie of your choice with either decaf coffee or tea

Lunch: grilled fish or tofu, mixed greens, and one serving of nuts and/or seeds

Dinner: carrot ginger soup and your choice of side salad

Snack options: This week choose one piece (or 1/2 cup) of fresh fruit, sliced raw vegetables (avoid sweet vegetables like carrots or beets this week) and/or one serving of any non-sweet snack found in the snack recipes section. To achieve the best fat loss results, limit snack foods to 300 calories for less. Do you best to consume 64-80 ounces of water today while keeping your sodium intake to 2,000 mg total or less.

Closing Thoughts

I'm not sure why we all get pulled into the tornado of what we think life is supposed to be about instead of accepting what it actually is. It typically takes years for us to realize that our stress, trauma and neglect are breeding grounds for our dis-ease. By the time we're middle aged, most of us are sadder than we should be, stricken with aches and pains and living much smaller lives than we want to live.

I am here to tell you that it doesn't have to be that way. We can be healthy, happy and whole human beings capable of enjoying every adventure that life has to offer, but that takes us learning how to take care of our physical, mental, spiritual and emotional health. It takes us tapping into who we are, what we want and like the NIKE tagline, we must "JUST DO IT."

The Detox Life is a strategy book designed to help you take control over your mindset, eat better, feel better and ultimately live better. As your coach, I'm encouraging you to be kind and flexible with yourself. I am encouraging you to let go of those things that no longer serve you so that you can nurture and promote the things that do. Every moment is a new opportunity for improvement, and now is the time to implement your plan of action. After all, this is the only life that you have, so you might as well take control start living it! If you should ever need my help digitally or in person, DO contact me at metralundycoaching@gmail.com.

"I believe that you are a valuable person within the collective humanity puzzle. What you choose to do or don't do affects everyone around you. Make positive change for yourself, your community and the world."

METRA LUNDY

APPENDIX

WATCH POWERFUL AND INSPIRING MOVIES

- **The Pursuit of Happiness** with Will Smith, Thandie Newton, Brian Howe

- **Creed I and II** with Tony Bellew, Richie Coster, Jacob and Michael B. Jordan, Sylvester Stallone, Tessa Thompson

- **Rocky** Sylvester Stallone, Talia Shire, Burt Young

- **McFarland, USA** with Kevin Costner, Maria Bello, Morgan Saylor

- **Remember the Titans** Denzel Washington, Will Patton, Donald Faison

- **A League of their Own** Lori Petty, Tom Hanks, Garry Marshall

- **Wonder Woman** Gal Gadot, Chris Pine, Robin Wright

- **The Miracle Worker: The Helen Keller Story** with Anne Bancroft, Patty Duke

- **To the Bone** with Lilly Collins

- **Unbroken** with Jack O'Connell, Domhnall Gleeson, and Miyavi

- **Hidden Figures** with Taraji P. Henson, Octavia Spencer and Janelle Monáe

- **Collateral Beauty** with Will Smith, Edward Norton, Keira Knightley

- **42: The Story of Jackie Robinson**

- **Without Limits** with Steve Prefontaine and Bill Bowerman

- **Zion** an Inspirational Short Film about Zion Clark

READ OR LISTEN TO POWERFUL AND INSPIRING BOOKS/AUDIOBOOKS

INSPIRING BOOKS

- **Can't Hurt Me** by David Goggins
- **Extreme Ownership** by Jacko Willink and Leif Babin
- **Man Up** by Bedros Keulian
- **Awaken the Giant Within** by Tony Robbins
- **Life In Motion: An Unlikely Ballerina** by Misty Copeland
- **In the Mean Time** Iyanla Vanzant
- **Relentless** by Tim Grover
- **The Power of Habit** by Charles Duhigg
- **The Foundation for Successful Change** by Zig Ziggler
- **The Art of Exceptional Living** by Jim Rohn
- **Living from Your Center: Guided Meditations for Creating Balance and Inner Strength** by Iyanla Vanzant

TAKE A DETOXIFYING BATH

Soak in soothing baths for 20-30 minutes or as long as it feels comforting. If you should feel light headed or nauseous do get out of the tub.

Recipe inspired by www.wellnessmama.com

SOOTHING SALT BATH

Ingredients

- 1/2 cup Sea Salt
- 1/2 cup Epsom Salt
- 1/2 cup Baking Soda
- 1/4 cup White Vinegar
- 2-10 drops of Peppermint or Eucalyptus Essential Oil *optional

Directions

In a dry container thoroughly mix dry ingredients; only then add contents to your warm bath.

Add wet ingredients to follow and enjoy!

HERBAL MINT BATH

Ingredients

- 1/4 cup of dried mint leaves
- 1/4 cup of dried chamomile
- 1-2 loose tea sachets

Directions

Add the dry ingredients to 1-2 loose tea sachets then add the sachets to your warm bath and enjoy!

CLAY BATH

Ingredients

- 1/2 cup Bentonite Clay
- 1/2 cup Epsom Salt
- 2-10 drops pure lemon essential oil *optional

Directions

Dissolve Epsom salt into a warm bath.

Using a wooden or glass container, mix bentonite clay with water and stir with a wooden or plastic spoon until mixture is smooth. Then add it to the bath water with the Epsom Salt.

Add essential oil if desired and enjoy!

FOOD REGIMEN DURING YOUR DETOXIFICATION

WHAT TO EAT

What you eat during your detoxification is extremely important. A healthy nutrient dense food regimen makes up more than half of the detox success picture. Success for each participant will vary but in general detoxifications should lead to you feeling lighter, more energetic, able bodied, disciplined and self-care conscious. For those reasons I highly recommend you working to improve on your normal diet. I've included a few options for eating below (in no particular order); remember that the best option takes you out of your comfort zone but gets you to your goals safely and gently. I encourage you to choose the level that nurtures you most.

- **Level Pescatarian** a person who does not eat meat but does eat fish and other shell foods

- **Level Lacto Ovo Vegetarian**: a vegetarian who consumes some animal products including but not limited to eggs and dairy

- **Level Vegetarian** a person who does not eat meat, seafood, the flesh of any animal but may consume foods that contain animal by-products

- **Level Vegan**: a person who strictly adheres to not consuming meats of any kind or foods with animal by-products

- **Level Vegan Rawtarian** a person who does not eat meat nor consume animal by-products. They maintain a one-hundred percent plant-based diet consuming foods in their raw state only. vegetables. Foods considered to be "raw", are ones who's average temperature does not exceed 115-118 degrees Fahrenheit.

HOW TO EAT

During your detoxification eat simple, unpackaged fresh foods that are mostly plants preferably prepared at home. If you have to consume packaged foods, do eat those foods with the fewest number of ingredients, sugar and sodium. If boredom becomes an issue, remember that variety will help you remain committed. Plan for meals that include lots of color, fresh herbs and spices.

WHEN TO EAT

Detoxing is a journey. Like everything else in your life, the more consistent you are with your diet, exercise and healthy living, the more likely you will see desirable results. That being said, I encourage you to eat on a schedule; you will be better able to access your body's responses to your lifestyle changes. Below I have given you options for scheduled eating using intermittent fasting as a centerpiece. I love this as a potential plan because it allows you to cycle through periods of fasting with no food and periods of eating when it works for you. I've included sample intermittent fasting schedules below. Please note that fasting schedules are personal. The one you choose should be the one that fits best in your life. Do make adjustments as needed.

- **14-10** (14 hours of fasting, 10 hours of eating) Example stop eating by 7 PM and resume eating by 9AM the following day

- **16-8** (16 hours of fasting, 8 hours of eating) Example stop eating by 7 PM and resume eating the following day by 11 AM *Recommended

- **18-6** (18 hours of fasting, 6 hours of eating) Example stop eating by 7 PM and resume eating the following day by 1PM

- **20-4** (20 hours of fasting, 4 hours of eating) Example stop eating by 7 PM and resume eating by 3 PM the following day

WHERE TO EAT DURING

Everything matters including where you consume your food. Support your body's healthy digestion by choosing to eat in places that encourage a sense of peace and calm.

WHY EAT DIFFERENTLY

Each time you engage in a detoxification you will evolve your state of living. Be sure to approach each detoxification knowing that if you desire a different personal outcome you will need to do something different to achieve that new outcome.

CALORIE COUNTING

A calorie is a unit of energy defined by the amount of heat required to raise 1 gram of water 1 degrees Celsius. In The Detox Life, when I talk about calories, I am talking about what you will need to sustain your body while helping you maintain and/or lose weight. If weight loss is your goal, plan to use up more calories (energy) than you consume. A great goal would be for you to burn 250-500 calories daily via exercise routine.

When your personal goals include losing weight or toning up, counting food calories helps tremendously. I am an advocate of counting calories because:

- You will be more aware of mindless eating

- Logging/tracking can be done by anyone, anytime and anywhere

- 5 popular calorie counting websites are

  » My Fitness Pal
  » Lose it!
  » FatSecret
  » Cron-O-Meter
  » SparkPeople

An emphasis on tracking will lead to greater personal accountability

- Calorie counting does not require expensive tests or tools

- Calorie information is present on most nutrition packaging

CONSUME THESE "EMBRACE FOODS" BASED ON YOUR CHOSEN LEVEL

Inspired by www.southbeachdiet.com

Consider this: All four weeks of your detox, make sure you stay hydrated! Your water intake should be equal to half of your body weight in ounces.

Note regarding seafood: Do limit your consumption of fish high in mercury and other contaminants including but not limited to marlin, swordfish, shark, tilefish, orange roughy, king mackerel, bigeye and ahi tuna, and canned albacore tuna (use light tuna instead).

- Fish (all types)
- Fish oil
- Tuna, water-packed light in cans or pouches, and other water-packed fish

DAIRY

Dairy is a known inflammatory food – eat it cautiously.

- Buttermilk, light (1.5%) (up to 2 one-cup servings daily)
- Evaporated milk, fat-free (up to one 2 tbsp. serving daily)
- Greek yogurt, nonfat (0%) plain (up to 2 one-cup servings daily)
- Half-and-half (up to one 2 tbsp. serving daily)
- Kefir, nonfat and low-fat plain (up to 2 one-cup servings daily)
- Milk, fat-free or 1% nonfat dry milk powder (up to 2 one-cup servings daily)

- Yogurt, nonfat or low-fat plain (up to 2 one-cup servings daily)
- Eggs (up to three eggs daily). Do consult with your healthcare professional with questions and/or concerns

SOY-BASED MEAT SUBSTITUTES AND MEAT ALTERNATIVES

Keep in mind that gluten is a known inflammatory food that can be found in bread, cereal pasta, soy meat alternatives – eat it cautiously. (Unless otherwise stated, look for products that have 6 g or less fat per 2-3 oz. serving)

- Seitan
- Soy bacon
- Soy burger
- Soy chicken, unbreaded
- Soy crumbles, 1/4 cup (2 oz.) suggested serving size (plain or seasoned)
- Soy hot dogs
- Soy sausage patties and tempeh links, 1/4 cup suggested serving size
- Tofu (all varieties), 1/2 cup suggested serving size
- Yuba (bean curd in sticks or sheets)

MILK SUBSTITUTES

- Soy milk, low-fat, unsweetened or low-sugar plain or vanilla (4 g or less fat per 8 oz. serving); or artificially sweetened soy milk (4 g or less fat per 8 oz. serving). Avoid products that contain high-fructose corn syrup.
- Almond milk, unsweetened, all flavors
- Coconut milk, unsweetened

BEANS AND OTHER LEGUMES

Fresh, dried, frozen, or canned (without added sugar). Start with a 1/3 to 1/2 – cup serving size. Use reduced-sodium canned products when available and wash the beans thoroughly before consuming them.

- Adzuki beans
- Black beans
- Black-eyed peas
- Broad beans
- Butter beans
- Cannellini beans
- Chickpeas (garbanzos)
- Hummus (2 oz.)
- Cranberry beans
- Edamame
- Fava beans
- Great Northern beans
- Italian beans
- Kidney beans
- Lentils (any variety)
- Lima beans
- Mung beans
- Navy beans
- Pigeon peas
- Pinto beans
- Refried beans, fat-free, canned
- Soybeans
- Split peas
- White beans

VEGETABLES

Eat as many fresh, unprocessed foods as possible. The general goal is to choose a more plant – based food regimen. When fresh food is not available you may use frozen or canned without added sugar. Do eat a vegetable with every meal.

- Artichoke hearts
- Artichokes
- Arugula
- Asparagus
- Bok choy
- Broccoli
- Broccolini
- Broccoli rabe
- Brussels sprouts
- Cabbage (green, red, napa, Savoy)
- Capers
- Cauliflower
- Celeriac (celery root)
- Celery
- Chayote
- Collard greens
- Cucumbers
- Daikon radishes
- Eggplant
- Endive
- Escarole
- Fennel
- Fiddlehead ferns
- Garlic
- Grape leaves
- Green beans
- Hearts of palm
- Jícama
- Kale

- Leeks
- Lettuce (all varieties)
- Mushrooms (all varieties)
- Mustard greens
- Okra
- Onions
- Parsley
- Peppers (all varieties)
- Pickles (avoid high-sodium or artificially sweetened)
- Pimientos
- Radicchio
- Radishes
- Rhubarb
- Sauerkraut
- Scallions
- Sea vegetables (avoid high-sodium seaweed nori)
- Shallots
- Snap peas
- Snow peas
- Spinach
- Sprouts (alfalfa, beans, broccoli, lentils, radish, sunflower)
- Squash, spaghetti
- Squash, summer
- Yellow Zucchini
- Swiss chard
- Tomatillos
- Tomatoes (fresh and all varieties of canned, jarred, and dried with 3 g of sugar or less per serving)
- Tomato juice, low-sodium
- Turnip greens
- Vegetable juice blends, low-sodium
- Water chestnuts
- Watercress
- Wax beans

NUTS AND SEEDS

Limit to one serving per day, as specified.

Always soak raw nuts for 24 hours prior to consuming.

- Almonds – 14
- Brazil nuts – 4
- Cashews – 15
- Chestnuts – 6
- Chia seeds – 3 Tbsp. (1 oz.)
- Coconut, unsweetened – 1/4 cup
- Edamame, dry roasted – 1/4 cup
- Filberts – 25 Flaxmeal (ground flaxseed) – 3 Tbsp.
- Flaxseed – 3 Tbsp. (1 oz.)
- Hazelnuts – 23
- Macadamias – 8
- Peanut butter, natural, and other nut butters (look for brands with 1 g of sugar or less per 2 Tbsp.) – 2 Tbsp.
- Pecans – 15
- Pine nuts (pignoli) – 1 oz.
- Pistachios – 30
- Pumpkin seeds – 3 Tbsp. (1 oz.)
- Sesame seeds – 3 Tbsp. (1 oz.)
- Soy nuts – 1/4 cup
- Sunflower seeds – 3 Tbsp. (1 oz.)
- Tahini – 2 Tbsp.
- Walnuts – 15

FATS/OILS

Up to 2 Tbsp. of the following fats or oils are allowed daily. Monounsaturated oils are particularly recommended.

Monounsaturated Oils:

- Canola
- Olive (particularly cold press extra-virgin)

Polyunsaturated Oils or a Blend of Monounsaturated and polyunsaturated:

- Corn
- Flaxseed
- Grapeseed
- Peanut
- Safflower
- Sesame
- Soybean
- Sunflower

Other Fats/Oils

- Avocado – 1/3 whole = 1 Tbsp. oil
- Coconut oil, extra-virgin – 1 Tbsp.
- Cream cheese substitute, dairy free – 2 Tbsp. (use occasionally)
- Guacamole – 1/2 cup = 1 Tbsp. oil
- Margarine, trans-fat-free – 2 Tbsp. (use only vegetable oil spread, not stick margarine)
- Mayonnaise, low-fat or light – 2 Tbsp. (avoid varieties made with high-fructose corn syrup)
- Mayonnaise, regular – 1 Tbsp.
- Olives (small green) 15 = 1/2 Tbsp. oil
- Olives (small black) 8 = 1/2 Tbsp. oil

- Salad dressing, prepared – 2 Tbsp. Use those that contain 3 g sugar or less per 2 Tbsp. Best choices contain canola or olive oil
- Sour cream, light and reduced-fat – 2 Tbsp. (use occasionally) Vegetable oil spread (margarine) – 2 Tbsp. Choose brands that do not contain trans fats
- Seasonings and Condiments
- All herbs and spices and herb and spice blends that contain no added sugar
- Arrowroot
- Broth of vegetables (preferably fat-free, low-sodium or less sodium)
- Chile peppers, fresh and dried
- Chile paste
- Chile sauce, sugar-free
- Chipotles in adobo
- Cocktail sauce, sugar-free
- Cooking sprays (such as olive oil, canola oil)
- Espresso powder
- Extracts (pure almond, vanilla, or others)
- Horseradish and horseradish sauce
- Hot pepper sauce
- Ketchup, sugar-free
- Lemon juice
- Lime juice
- Liquid smoke
- Mustard, all types, except honey mustard
- Pepper, ground and whole peppercorns (black, cayenne, pink, white, and pepper blends)
- Salsa (check label for added sugar)
- Vinegar, all types
- Wasabi, powdered or paste

TOPPINGS AND SAUCES

Use the following toppings and sauces sparingly; check label for added sugar or monosodium glutamate (MSG) and try to avoid them.

- Coconut milk canned lite (1/4 cup max.)
- Cream cheese, fat-free – 2 Tbsp.
- Miso – 1/2 Tbsp.
- Pesto sauce – 2 Tbsp.
- Nama Shoyu – 1/2 Tbsp.
- Sour cream, fat-free – 2 Tbsp.
- Soy sauce, reduced-sodium – 1/2 Tbsp.
- Sriracha sauce – 1 tsp.
- Steak sauce – 1/2 Tbsp.
- Taco sauce – 1 Tbsp.
- Tamari – 1 Tbsp.
- Tapenade — 2 Tbsp.
- Worcestershire sauce – 1 Tbsp.

STARCHES

Choose a small portion of one of these whole grains, and make sure you eat it before noon.

- 1/4 – 1/2 cup old fashioned or steel cut oatmeal
- 1/4 – 1/2 cup quinoa cooked

Sweet Treats

- Limit to 75-100 calories per day
- Chocolate powder, no sugar added
- Chocolate syrup, sugar-free
- Cocoa powder, unsweetened baking type, labeled 100% cacao
- Gelatin, sugar-free

- Gum, sugar-free
- Jams and jellies, sugar-free
- Pops, sugar-free Syrups, sugar-free

Sugar Substitutes

- Agave nectar (1 Tbsp. daily max.)
- Stevia - 1 Tbsp
- 100% Maple Syrup – 1 Tbsp
- Raw Honey – 1 Tbsp
- Sugar n the Raw – 1 Tbsp

Beverages

- Almond milk, unsweetened, all flavors (limit to 2 cups daily as part of total dairy servings)
- Caffeinated and decaffeinated coffee and tea (drink caffeinated in moderation)
- Club soda
- Coconut milk beverage, unsweetened (limit to 2 cups daily as part of total dairy servings)
- Herbal teas (peppermint, chamomile, etc.)
- Kefir, nonfat and low-fat plain
- Seltzer
- Soymilk, low-fat, unsweetened or low-sugar plain or vanilla (4 g or less fat per 8 oz. serving); or artificially sweetened soy milk (4 g or less fat per 8 oz. serving). Avoid products that contain high-fructose corn syrup. (Limit to 2 cups daily as part of total dairy servings.)
- Tomato juice, low-sodium
- Vegetable juice blends, low-sodium

AVOID FOODS

Limit sodium to no more than 2000mg daily.

Limit refined sweeteners including sugar, honey and agave to no more than 24g daily.

MEATS

- Beef (all types)
- Poultry (all types)
- Pork (all types)
- Game meats (all types)

DAIRY

- Ice cream
- Milk, 2% or whole
- Frozen yogurt
- Cheese

AVOID THESE FRUITS FOR THE FIRST TWO WEEKS OF YOUR DETOX

- Banana
- Pineapple
- Mango
- Papaya
- Grapes
- All melons (watermelon, cantaloupe, honey dew)

During weeks three and four, limit these fruits to 2 pieces or 1 cup per day for breakfast or lunch. Avoid at dinnertime.

AVOID THESE VEGETABLES FOR THE FIRST TWO WEEKS OF YOUR DETOX

- Beets
- Carrots
- Corn
- Green Peas
- Potatoes, Sweet
- Potatoes, White
- Pumpkin
- Squash, winter
- Turnips (root)
- Yams

STARCHES

- Bread, all types
- Processed cereals, all types
- Croutons, all types
- Matzo
- Pasta, all types
- Pastries and baked goods
- Rice, all types for the first two weeks of your detox

CONDIMENTS

- Cocktail sauce
- Ketchup

BEVERAGES

- Alcohol of any kind including beer and wine
- Processed fruit juices of all types; if consuming fresh juice, do respect the fruit intake recommendation and allowable serving amounts
- Powdered drink mixes containing sugar
- Soda and other drinks containing sugar
- Soy milk with more than 4g fat per 8 oz serving
- Sodas (diet or regular)

LOVE AND USE YOUR SPICES AND SUPPLEMENTS

1. BASIL ALSO CALLED SAINT-JOSEPH'S WORT

Common uses: teas and spices for food

Origins: Native to tropical regions of central Africa and Southeast Asia

Flavors: fragrant, pungent, mild to strong

Health benefits: high in vitamin K and A and beta-carotene; thought to aid in digestion and stress relief as well as lower cholesterol

Fun fact: from the Latin word basilius, meaning "royal". In ancient times, basil was considered sacred

2. BLACK PEPPER (UNRIPE DRIED BERRY OF FROM THE PIPER NIGRUM PLANT)

Common uses: spice for food

Origins: South Western India, Kerala

Flavors: spicy, medium to hot

Health benefits: contains important minerals such as chromium, calcium, copper, zinc, magnesium, manganese, and phosphorous. Also high in Vitamin K and beta-carotene; it works to improve digestion

Fun fact: all types of pepper spice white, black, green and red come from the same plant. The colors vary based on how ripe the berry is and the processed used to harvest it

3. CAROB ALSO KNOWN AS ST. JOHN'S BREAD, LOCUST BEAN OR LOCUST TREE

Common uses: food supplement or spice

Origins: North Africa and Southern Europe

Flavors: chocolaty

Health benefits: anti-inflammatory properties; high in anti-antioxidants, calcium, and fiber

Fun fact: is a flowering evergreen shrub

4. COCOA

Common uses: food supplement or spice

Origins: Native to the Amazon Basin

Flavors: chocolaty

Health benefits: rich in antioxidants and flavonoids

Fun fact: dried fruit of the fermented seed of the Theobroma cacao

5. CELERY SEED

Common uses: spice for food

Origins: Natively from: Europe and Asia

Flavors: earthy, grassy, and slightly bitter

Health benefits: flavonoids, antioxidants, linoleic acid and omega-6 fatty acid; thought to relieve stomach bloating, flatulence, indigestion and acts a diuretic

Fun fact: It takes just one once of celery seed to produce one acre of celery

6. CHIA SEEDS

Common uses: supplément

Origins: Mexico and Guatemala

Flavors: mild, nutty

Health benefits: high in zinc, omega-3 fatty acids, antioxidants and fiber. Seeds are thought to promote better digestion

Fun fact: Ancient Aztecs used chia seeds as a form of money

7. CHIVES

Common uses: teas and spice for food

Origins: Natively from Asia and Europe

Flavors: mild onion

Health benefits: rich in antioxidants, dietary fiber, B-complex vitamins, copper, iron, manganese, zinc and calcium.

Fun fact: First cultivated during the middle ages in Europe

8. CILANTRO (LEAVES)

Common uses: tea and spice for food

Origins: Southern Europe

Flavors: fragrant, mild to strong

Health benefits: high in Vitamin K; contains manganese and trace minerals; aides digestion and helps relieve symptoms of hypoglycemia such as dizziness, confusion, and fatigue

Fun fact: Ancient Egyptians were thought to use cilantro to cure urinary tract infections

9. CINNAMON

Common uses: teas and spice for food

Origins: Sri Lanka

Flavors: sweet, woody, aromatic

Health benefits: high in antioxidants, flavonoids, calcium and fiber; thought to be anti-inflammatory, prevent the clotting of blood and stimulate blood flow

Fun fact: At one time, cinnamon was worth more than the price of gold

10. CLOVES

Common uses: teas and spice for food

Origins: Madagascar, Indonesia and Sri Lanka

Flavors: pungent, strong, and sweet

Health benefits: anti-inflammatory, reduces inflammation and is a natural breath freshener

Fun fact: spice has also been smoked like a cigarette

11. CORIANDER SEEDS, ALSO KNOWN AS CILANTRO OR CHINESE PARSLEY

Common uses: spice for food

Origins: Iran

Flavors: tart, lemon/lime

Health benefits: high in Vitamins A and K, beta-carotene, calcium, manganese, potassium and iron

Fun fact: leaves are 92% water, 4% carbohydrate, 2% protein and less than 1% fat

12. CUMIN

Common uses: spice for food

Origins: Natively to India

Flavors: earthy, nutty

Health benefits: high in iron, dietary fiber and minerals; thought to reduce inflammation, aid in digestion and detoxification of the liver

Fun fact: Is a member of the parsley family

13. FENNEL

Common uses: teas and spices for food

Origins: North Africa, Southern Europe and Asia

Flavors: mild licorice

Health benefits: high in B-complex vitamins, phytonutrients and fiber; thought to reduce inflammation, promote a healthy blood pressure, reduce the risk of heart attack and strokes

Fun fact: Can grow to be up to five feet in high (60 inches)

14. GARLIC POWDER

Common uses: teas and spices for food

Origins: Central Asia and Northeastern Iran

Flavors: mild, sweet, stale

Health benefits: rich in potassium, iron, calcium, magnesium, manganese, zinc and selenium; thought to be anti-bacterial, anti-fungal and a great immune booster

Fun fact: garlic is closely related to the vegetables onion, chives, shallots and leeks

15. GINGER

Common uses: teas and spice for food

Origins: Southeast Asia

Flavors: fragrant, pungent mild to strong

Health benefits: high in antioxidants and properties that reduce inflammation; thought to aid in digestion

Fun fact: Can be harvested to produce a juice, powder or oil

16. LAVENDER

Common uses: teas and spice or garnish for food

Origins: Cape Verde, Canary Islands, Southern Europe, East Africa, Asia

Flavors: woody, floral, pungent with an undertone of mint

Health benefits: thought to have antiseptic calming effect and promote a relaxed state

Fun fact: Nectar makes great-quality honey

17. MINT

Common uses: teas and spices for food

Origins: Natively from Asia, North America, Southern Africa and Australia

Flavors: fragrant, fresh

Health benefits: thought to aid in digestion, relieve headache tension and soothe irritated skin

Fun fact: Ancient Romans believed that eating mint would increase intelligence

18. MISO PASTE

Common uses: spice for food

Origins: Japanese

Flavors: mild earthy

Health benefits: high in copper, manganese, Vitamin K, zinc phosphorus choline and essential amino acids; thought to be a great probiotic for the gut

Fun fact: a Japanese word meaning fermented beans

19. NUTMEG

Common uses: spice for food

Origins: Indonesia and the West Indies

Flavors: sweet, nutty

Health benefits: high in B-complex vitamins, Vitamin C, folic acid, riboflavin, niacin, Vitamin A and flavonoids; thought to be anti-fungal, antidepressant and great for digestion

Fun fact: seed kernel of the nutmeg fruit

20. NUTRITIONAL YEAST

Common uses: vegan flavoring

Flavors: cheesy, nutty

Health benefits: high in minerals selenium, iron and zinc; it is also a complete protein which means it contains the nine essential amino acids

Fun fact: made from a single celled organism called Saccaromyces Cerevisiae which is grown in molasses, harvested and dried in heat to deactivate

21. ONION POWDER

Common uses: spice for food

Origins: Central Asia

Flavors: strong, mild, aromatic

Health benefits: high in vitamins, minerals and antioxidants; thought promote heart health as well as prevent certain types of cancers

Fun fact: made from dehydrated ground onion; common ingredients seasoned salt and other spices

22. PAPRIKA

Common uses: spice for food

Origins: Mexico

Flavors: mild to hot

Health benefits: high in vitamin A, iron, and dietary fiber; contains carotenoids thought promote healthy eye function

Fun fact: made from the dried red fruit of the Capsicum annum plant also known as the bell pepper or sweet pepper

23. SAGE

Common uses: teas and spice for food

Origins: Mediterranean

Flavors: sweet and somewhat bitter

Health benefits: high in vitamin K, antioxidants and vitamin A; thought to aid in digestion, relieve abdominal cramping, bloating as well as be antibacterial

Fun fact: Latin name Salvia which means to save or heal

24. SEA SALT

Common uses: spice for food

Origins: Mediterranean

Flavors: salty

Health benefits: rich in minerals, sodium, potassium, calcium and magnesium; aids in sustaining hydration levels

Fun fact: made from evaporated sea water

25. SPIRULINA

Common uses: supplement

Origins: Africa and Mexico

Flavors: fishy, depending on the brand used

Health benefits: high in antioxidants, minerals, fiber and amino acids

Fun fact: gets its name because it comes from a spiral-like bacteria called cyanobacteria

26. STEVIA

Common uses: teas and sweetener

Origins: Natively from Asia

Flavors: bitter, sweet

Health benefits: studies show that it may help control blood sugar and insulin

Fun fact: offers roughly 40 times more sweetness than sugar but has almost zero calories

27. TAHINI

Common uses: supplement for food

Origins: North Africa

Flavors: nutty

Health benefits: high in iron, thiamin, phosphorus and magnesium; thought to maintain healthy bones

Fun fact: made from sesame seeds that are hulled, ground and toasted

28. TARRAGON

Common uses: teas and spice for food

Origins: Russia and Western Asia

Flavors: fragrant, slightly bitter

Health benefits: rich in potassium and Vitamin A; thought to neutralize the effects of free radicals as well as help increase muscle creatine absorption

Fun fact: has historically been used to relieve toothaches

29. TURMERIC

Common uses: teas and spice for food

Origins: Natively from Asia

Flavors: bitter, earthy

Health benefits: rich in antioxidants, flavonoids, omega-3 fatty acids; thought to reduce inflammation, regulator of blood sugar levels and blood fat levels

Fun fact: Primary ingredient in many commercial sunscreens

30. WHEATGRASS

Common uses: supplement

Origins: North America and Europe

Flavors: earthy

Health benefits: rich in chlorophyll, amino acids, minerals, vitamins and enzymes

Fun fact: new leaves of the common wheat plant

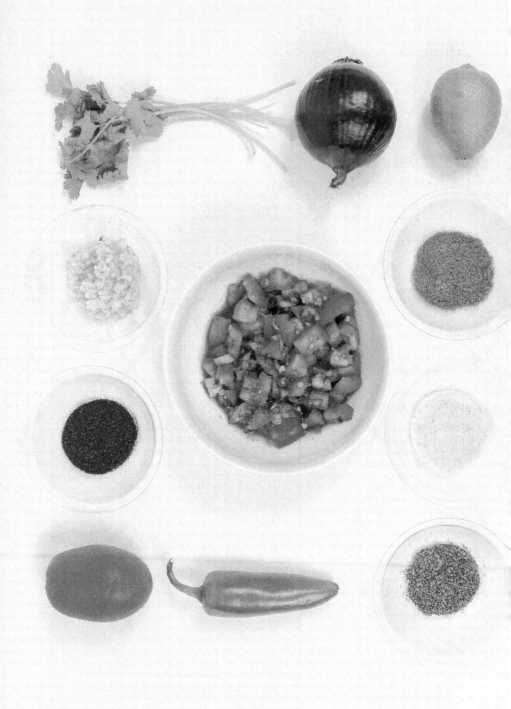

RECIPES

FRESH FRUIT AND VEGETABLE JUICE RECIPES

It is best to drink juice immediately or within 15 minutes of blending

1. TANGY MAMACITA - JUICE OR BLEND

Serves 1-2

Ingredients
- 1/2 lime
- 1 orange
- 1/2 cup pineapple
- 1 cup romaine lettuce
- 1/2 teaspoon wheatgrass
- 1/2 teaspoon spirulina
- 1/4 - 1/2 cup of water

Directions
1. using a knife, remove the skin from the lime, lemon, orange and pineapple; lightly rinse pulp and add to a high speed blender or juicer
2. rinse romaine lettuce and add to blender or juicer as well
3. spoon in spirulina and wheatgrass
4. add water and enjoy *add more water to dilute sweetness

2. GQ (GREEN QUEEN) - BLEND

Inspired by Heal Thyself Natural Living Cookbook
Serves 1-2

Ingredients
- 2 cups water
- 1 teaspoon spirulina
- 1 teaspoon wheatgrass
- 1/4 cup chopped curly parsley
- 1/2 lemon
- 1 teaspoon of raw honey *optional

Directions
1. using a knife, remove the skin of the lemon and add pulp to a high speed blender
2. rinse parsley and add to blender
3. spoon in spirulina, wheatgrass and honey
4. blend with water and enjoy

3. AUTUMN SPICE - JUICE

Serves 1-2

Ingredients
- 2 carrots
- 1 medium red apple peeled
- 1 1/2 inch piece of ginger
- 1/4 lemon
- pinch of cinnamon
- pinch of ground cloves
- 1 cup of water

Directions

1. scrape the outside of the carrot to remove the outer layer of skin; cut into small pieces and add to a juicer
2. slice apple and discard the core; add to juicer
3. remove the skin of the lemon and ginger and add to the juicer
4. add cloves and cinnamon
5. let juice sit for 1-2 minutes then enjoy

4. BERRY FUNNY - BLEND

Serves 1-2

Ingredients

- 1/2 cup strawberries
- 1/2 cup watermelon
- 1/4 lime
- 2 cups butter lettuce
- 1/2 - 1 cup water

Directions

1. add strawberries, watermelon and lettuce to a high speed blender
2. remove the skin from the lime, and add pulp to blender
3. use water to blend ingredients and enjoy

5. HEAVENLY CELERY JUICE

Serves 1-2

Ingredients

- 8-10 celery stalks juiced
- 1/4 cup water

Directions

1. add rinsed celery stalks to a juicer
2. mix with water
3. enjoy

6. SPRING SONG - BLEND OR JUICE

Serves 1-2

Ingredients

- 1 grapefruit
- 1/2 lemon
- 1 orange
- 1/4-1/2 cup of fresh mint water
- 1 cup of baby spinach

Directions

1. to make fresh mint water add 1 cup of water to a saucepan with a 1/4 cup of fresh mint leaves in a tea sachet. bring to a boil then steep for 5-10 minutes. refrigerate extra for later use
2. remove the skin from grapefruit, lemon and orange and add pulp to a high speed blender or juicer
3. then add fresh mint and spinach
4. mix with water and enjoy

7. CUCUMBER COOLER JUICE

Serves 1-2

Ingredients

- 1 large cucumber peeled
- 1 red apple
- 1/4 cup fresh mint water

Directions

1. remove the skin from the cucumber and apple and add pulp to a juicer
2. then add water
3. enjoy

8. BANANA BABY BLEND

Serves 1-2

Ingredients

- 1 ripe banana
- 1/4 cup of sweet strawberries
- 1/2 avocado
- 1 cup baby spinach
- 1/2 - 1 cup of water

Directions

1. remove the skin from the banana and avocado and add pulp to a high speed blender
2. then add baby spinach and strawberries
3. blend with water and enjoy

9. APPARENTLY DELIGHTFUL - BLEND

Serves 1-2

Ingredients

- 1 red apple
- 1 sweet pear
- 1 cup baby kale
- 1/2 - 1 cup of water

Directions

1. remove the skin from the apple and pear if not organic; cut up and add to a high speed blender
2. then add kale
3. blend with water and enjoy

10. GK (GREEN KING) - BLEND

Inspired by Heal Thyself Natural Living Cookbook
Serves 1-2

Ingredients

- 2 cups baby spinach
- 1 medium cucumber
- 4 Tablespoon chopped watercress
- 4 Tablespoons chopped curly parsley
- 1 carrot
- 1-2 sprigs of thyme
- 1/2 cup of water

Directions

1. remove the skin from the cucumber; cut up and add to high speed blender
2. scrape the outer layer of the carrot; cut up and add to blender
3. then add spinach, watercress, parsley and thyme
4. blend with water and enjoy

11. SUMMER BREEZE BLEND

Serves 1-2

Ingredients
- 1/2 cup of water
- 1/2 cup honey dew
- 1/4 lime
- 1 cup baby romaine lettuce

Directions
1. remove the skin from the lime and honeydew and add pulp to a high speed blender
2. then add lettuce and mint water
3. blend and enjoy

12. CHOCOLATE PROTEIN SMOOTHIE BLEND

Serves 1-2

Ingredients
- 2-3 pitted dates soak for 10 minutes; blend first
- 1/4 cup natural unsalted sunflower seeds
- 1/4 cup of cashews *soak for 24 hours
- 2-3 Tablespoons cacao powder
- 1 cup unsweetened non-dairy coconut yogurt
- 1 - 1 1/2 cup of water
- 1 cup baby spinach

Directions
1. measure out and soak cashews head of time
2. add all other ingredients to a blender and enjoy

13. VANILLA PROTEIN SMOOTHIE BLEND

Serves 1-2

Ingredients

- 1 large peach
- 1 whole avocado
- 1-2 pitted dates soak for 10 minutes; blend first
- 1/4 natural unsalted pumpkin seeds
- 1 cup baby spinach
- 1/4 teaspoon vanilla extract
- 1 cup unsweetened non-dairy coconut yogurt
- 1/4 cup of water

Directions

1. remove skin from peach; cut up and freeze
2. once frozen add to high speed blender
3. then add all other ingredients and enjoy

BREAKFAST

1. BREAKFAST BENTO BOX

Serves 1

Ingredients
- 1/4 cup strawberries
- 1/4 cup blueberries
- 2 Tablespoons sweet cashew cream
- 3 almond crackers
- 2 raw celery stalks cut into 3 inch pieces
- 1/4 cup sesame Asian no-fry stir fry*see recipe in salad section
- 1 Tablespoon almond butter with a drizzle of raw agave

Directions
1. place berries in a container together and spoon in sweet cashew cream
2. add agave drizzled almond butter to almond crackers
3. place celery and sesame stir-fry on plate and add almond smothered crackers
4. enjoy

2. WAKE'M UP OVERNIGHT OATS

Serves 1

Ingredients
- 1/2 cup old fashion rolled oats
- 2 teaspoons 100% maple syrup
- 1/8 teaspoon sea salt*optional
- 2/3 – 3/4 unsweetened almond milk
- 1/2 teaspoon vanilla extract

- 1 teaspoon almond slices *optional
- 1/4 cacao nibs *optional

Directions
1. place all ingredients in mason jar or other sealable container
2. allow them to sit overnight
3. oats can be eaten cold or heated once done
4. top with almond slices and cacao nibs
5. enjoy

3. CREAM OF QUINOA

Serves 1

Ingredients
- 1/4 cup quinoa cooked
- 1/4 cup old fashion rolled oats
- 1/4 cup unsweetened almond milk
- 2 teaspoons raw agave
- 1 – 1 1/2 cup water

Directions
1. add quinoa and oats to a saucepan with water. Simmer for 20 minutes or until quinoa is soft and fluffy
2. remove quinoa and oat mixture from saucepan to a bowl
3. add all other ingredients
4. cool and enjoy

4. CARIBBEAN CURRY VEGETABLES AND TOFU

Recipe by www.thejamaicanmother.com
Serves 4-6

Ingredients

- 2 cups extra firm tofu drained and pat down to dry
- 15 ounce can chickpeas or from dried chickpeas
- 3 Tablespoons curry powder
- 3 small Yukon potatoes
- 3 medium carrots
- 1 medium onion
- 1/4 green pepper
- 1/4 yellow pepper
- 1/4 red pepper
- 1/4 Scotch Bonnet bell pepper
- 3 cloves garlic
- 1 teaspoon cornstarch
- Pinch salt
- Pinch black pepper
- 1 Tablespoon olive oil

Directions Curry Vegetables

1. boil soy chunks in water for 10 minutes. Remove from water, allow them to drain in a strainer
2. petite chop potatoes, carrots, bell peppers, onion and Scotch Bonnet pepper
3. boil potatoes and carrots for 10 minutes
4. in another pot add olive oil, onion, peppers, garlic, salt, pepper, and cornstarch. then add curry powder to pot
5. stir in chickpeas and cook on low for fifteen minutes. Stir often then add water allow ingredients to simmer for another fifteen minutes
6. once done, add potatoes, carrots and tofu chunks
7. mix well and simmer for another fifteen minutes on low heat
8. allow ingredients to cool
9. enjoy

5. BASIC VEGAN OR ORGANIC EGG OMELET

by www.blog.fatfreevegan.com
Serves 1-2

Ingredients Vegan Omelet

- 1/2 package of firm silken tofu
- 1 Tablespoon unsweetened soymilk
- 1 Tablespoon nutritional yeast
- 1 Tablespoon cornstarch
- 1/8 teaspoon onion powder
- 1/8 teaspoon turmeric
- 1/4 teaspoon salt
- 1/4 teaspoon black pepper
- pinch smoked paprika
- 1 cup of your favorite vegetables of choice for filling *optional

Directions Vegan Omelet

1. using a high speed blender, blend all ingredients together
2. add a dab of oil to a frying pan
3. pour the batter into the pan so that it makes a circular patty about 6-8 inches across the pan. *add your favorite vegetables of choice for filling
4. use a spatula to smooth over the top then cover
5. allow batter to cook at low heat for 3-5 minutes until batter edges have dried out and the middle is no longer a liquid
6. using a spatula lift one side of the omelet to see if it is set. It should be golden brown in color.
7. once ready use your spatula to fold one edge of the omelet over the other
8. cook for another minute then carefully slide omelet onto a plate
9. allow it to cool
10. enjoy

Ingredients Organic Egg Omelet

- 2 organic cage free eggs
- 4 Tablespoon unsweetened nut milk of choice
- 1 Tablespoon nutritional yeast
- 1/8 teaspoon onion powder
- 1/8 teaspoon turmeric
- 1/4 teaspoon salt
- 1/4 teaspoon black pepper
- pinch smoked paprika
- 1 cup of your favorite vegetables of choice for filling *optional

Directions

1. whisk together eggs and milk
2. add nutritional yeast, onion powder, turmeric, salt, pepper and paprika to eggs
3. add a dab of oil to a frying pan
4. pour the batter into the pan so that it makes a circular patter about 6-8 inches across the pan. *add your favorite vegetables of choice for filling
5. use a spatula to smooth over the top then cover
6. allow batter to cook at low heat for 3-5 minutes until batter edges have dried out and the middle is no longer a liquid
7. using a spatula lift one side of the omelet to see if it is set. It should be golden brown in color.
8. once ready use your spatula to fold one edge of the omelet over the other
9. cook for another minute then carefully slide omelet onto a plate
10. allow it to cool
11. enjoy

LUNCH OR DINNER
ENTRÉE RECIPES

1. COLLARD GREEN BURRITO

Recipe by www.minimalistbaker.com
Serves 4

Walnut Filling
- 3 cups walnuts
- 2/3 cups sun dried tomatoes soaked
- 4 cloves garlic minced
- 1/2 Sea salt
- 1 Tablespoon smoked paprika
- 1 Tablespoon ground cumin
- 1 Tablespoon chili powder
- 1-2 Habanera peppers deseeded
- 2 teaspoons nutritional yeast
- 1/4 cup water

Topping
- 2 Tablespoons cashew sour cream
- 2 Tablespoons per burrito fresh homemade salsa
- 1/2 ripe avocado
- 1/4 teaspoon hot sauce *optional
- 1 cup Alfalfa sprouts
- 1 Tablespoon pickled red onion
- 1/4 - 1/2 cup water
- 1 Tablespoon apple cider vinegar
- 1 Tablespoon lemon juice
- 1/4 cup red cabbage

Shell
- 4 large collard greens

Directions walnut meat
1. put walnuts in food processor and process until finely chopped
2. add remaining ingredients to the food processor and mix well
3. spoon all ingredients into a bowl and set aside for later use

Directions for topping
1. prepare cashew sour cream according to recipe*see section on sauces and dressing
2. prepare homemade salsa according to recipe *see section on sauces and dressings
3. remove skin of avocado, slice into medium size pieces and set aside
4. gently rinse alfalfa sprouts and set aside
5. slice 1 whole red onion and set in enough water to cover them by one inch. Pour in apple cider vinegar and lemon juice. Allow this to sit for 30 minutes

Directions for burrito
1. place collard green on a cutting board or plate. Remove the thickest stalk at the bottom of the leaf for easy folding
2. vertically add walnut mixture down the center vein of the green
3. top walnuts mixture with pickled red cabbage, red onion, avocado, hot sauce, sour cream and alfalfa sprouts
4. when done, close the burrito by folding in the short edges first then the long ones
5. flip the burrito so that the folded edges are down
6. cut down the middle to half the burrito
7. enjoy

2. CREAMY MUSHROOM SAUCE AND SQUASH NOODLES ENTRÉE

Serves 3

Ingredients Squash Noodles
- 3 large yellow squash spiralized
- 1/2 teaspoon pink Himalayan salt

Ingredients and Directions Mushroom sauce
- *see under section on sauces and dressings

Directions Squash noodles
1. peel outer layer of squash noodles off and discard
2. using a spiralizer put turn each squash into to squash noodles
3. add noodles to a colander
4. spoon in salt, gently massage and allow noodles to sit. They will drain excess water and taste even more like noodles
5. once done add noodles to a plate and set aside

Directions on Entrée
1. take 1 1/2 cups of squash noodles and add to a plate
2. then spoon on mushroom sauce *the sauce could be served hot or at room temperature
3. top sauce with 2 Tablespoons of mushrooms
4. add more salt and pepper to taste and Enjoy

3. ZOODLE MAC AND CHEESE

Serves 3

Ingredients Zucchini Noodles
- 4 medium zucchini noodles spiralized
- Ingredients and Directions Mac and Cheese sauce
- *see under section on sauces and dressings

Directions Zucchini noodles
1. peel outer layer of squash noodles off and discard of the skin
2. using a spiralizer turn each zucchini into a zucchini noodles aka zoodle
3. once done add noodles to a plate and set aside

Directions on Entrée
1. take 1 1/2 cups of zoodles and add to a plate
2. then spoon on mac and cheese sauce *the sauce could be served hot or at room temperature
3. mix well
4. enjoy

4. STUFFED CABBAGE

Recipe by www.theveglife.com
Serves 4

Ingredients sauce
- 28 ounce can diced tomatoes
- 6 ounce can tomato paste
- 1 cup vegetable broth
- 1 small onion diced
- 1 teaspoon agave

- 1/2 cup non-dairy creamer *example So Delicious Coconut Original Creamer
- pinch salt
- pinch pepper
- 1 Tablespoon "Vegan Can't Believe It's Not Butter" *use vegan butter option/it's okay if it's a different brand

Ingredients roll
- 1 medium cabbage
- 1 cup veggie crumbles*choose your favorite brand
- 1/2 cup brown rice
- 1/4 cup onion petite diced and sautéed
- pinch salt
- pinch pepper

Directions sauce
1. melt butter in a saucepan and sauté onions until translucent to light brown
2. add diced tomatoes with the juice, vegetable stock, salt and pepper
3. then add tomatoes paste and taste in order to adjust seasonings. Add agave to balance out the tart taste created by the tomato paste
4. allow sauce to simmer for 30 minutes then add creamer. Simmer again for another 15 minutes

5. directions rolls
1. partially boil the head of cabbage just enough to easily peel cabbage layers apart. Do not overcook. The leave should be crisp but pliable. If you remove the core of the cabbage it will be easier to remove peel the cabbage layers apart
2. in a bowl mix the roll ingredients. Then spoon in a 1/2 cup of the sauce to help keep the mixture together
3. then take the roll filling and place it in the center of a cabbage leaf. Make sure to not overstuff the leaf

4. roll the ends of the stuffed cabbage and close with a toothpick. Do this until either the cabbage or cabbage filling is gone. Remember to remove the toothpick when serving
5. place finished rolls into a large saucepan or crock pot stacking them largest at the bottom to smallest at the top
6. add the sauce to the pot covering the rolls. Add more vegetable broth of the pot you needed
7. simmer cabbage rolls for 1 hour allowing the cabbage to look translucent and the filling is hot inside. Once done let cabbage rolls sit for 10 minutes
8. plate
9. enjoy

5. MEATLESS MEATLOAF

Recipe by www.simpleveganblog.com
Serves 6-8

Ingredients Meatloaf
- 1 cup canned or cooked chickpeas drained and rinsed
- 1 cup canned or cooked kidney beans drained and rinsed
- 1 cup ground flaxseed
- 1 cup nutritional yeast
- 1/2 cup tahini
- 1/4 cup Nama Shoya or tamari
- 1/4 cup unsweetened plant milk of choice
- 2 teaspoons onion powder
- 2 teaspoons garlic powder
- 1/4 teaspoon black pepper

Ingredients Glaze
- 1/2 cup ketchup
- 1/2 teaspoon agave
- 1 teaspoon onion powder

- 1 teaspoon garlic powder
- 1/2 teaspoon paprika

Directions
1. preheat oven to 350 degrees F
2. add chickpeas and beans to a bowl; mash together
3. add all other ingredients to chickpea and bean mash and mix well
4. press mash into a 9x5 inch loaf pan and form loaf shape with your hands
5. make glaze by mixing glaze ingredients in a bowl
6. spread the glaze over the top of the loaf and bake for 50 minutes
7. remove from the oven and allow it to cool
8. then plate, slice and Enjoy

6. CARIBBEAN ESCOVITCH FISH

Recipe by www.caribbeanpot.com
Serves 2

Ingredients fish
- 1 red snapper
- 1 scallion or green onion
- 3 sprigs thyme
- 1/4 teaspoon salt
- 1/4 teaspoon black pepper
- 1 fresh lime

Sauce
- 3/4 cup vinegar
- 1/4 teaspoon allspice
- 1 large onion
- 1 carrot
- 1 green pepper

- 1/2 Scotch Bonnet pepper *remove the seeds/create hot spice
- pinch salt 1/2 teaspoon agave

Directions for fish
1. Rinse fish with water then squeeze on fresh lime. Rinse again and allow the water to drain off
2. Rub the fish with spices salt, pepper and set aside
3. Add olive oil to a frying pan and heat the oil
4. Then add seasoned fish to the non-stick frying pan and place thyme on top. Allow fish to cook 4-5 minutes then flip the fish to the other side for more cooking. It's okay to move the thyme around the pot
5. Once done add the fish to paper towel to soak up any excess oil. Set the fish aside

Directions for sauce and fish
1. add all other ingredients to a saucepan and simmer until vegetables are crunchy to lightly soft about 3-4 minutes
2. place fish on a platter, pour sauce onto the fish and enjoy

7. VEGAN EGGPLANT PARMESAN

Recipe by www.minimalistbaker.com
Serves 2-3

Ingredients and Directions Marinara Sauce*see sauce recipe
- 2 cups marinara sauce

Ingredients Eggplant Parmesan
- 1 medium eggplant
- 1/4 cup almond flour
- 1 cup finely ground old fashion oats
- 2 Tablespoons vegan parmesan or nutritional yeast
- 1 teaspoon dried oregano

- 1/4 teaspoon sea salt
- 1/2 cup of unsweetened almond milk
- 1 teaspoon cornstarch

Directions Eggplant Parmesan

1. slice eggplant into thin rounds slightly less than 1/2 inch thick
2. sprinkle each side of eggplant with salt then arrange in a colander and sit colander in the sink. This process will help draw out the bitter taste of the eggplant
3. once done, let eggplant rest for 15 minutes. Then arrange each eggplant piece onto a clean absorbent dish towel. When that is done, place another absorbent dish towel on top of the eggplant pieces. Then add a baking sheet or heavy pan on top of the towel to help press out any additional water from the eggplant for 10 minutes
4. preheat oven to 400 degrees F
5. coat a baking sheet with a light spray of oil and set aside
6. prepare eggplant dipping stations – mix almond milk and cornstarch in a bowl and set aside; add flour to another bowl and finely ground oats, salt, oregano and vegan parmesan mixture to a third bowl
7. once the eggplant is thoroughly dried dip each piece as follows: (1) flour bowl, (2) almond milk bowl (3) oats bowl
8. arrange on baking sheet and bake for 20-30 minutes
9. coat a frying pan in olive oil and heat oil. Add 2-3 pieces of eggplant to the oil to sauté until light brown then remove from the pan onto a paper towel
10. allow eggplant to cool and enjoy *eggplant can be eaten with veggie noodles, coated with marinara sauce and garnished with parsley

8. MEATLESS MEATBALLS

Recipe by www.wholefully.com
Serves 4-6

Meatless Meatballs
- 1 14oz. can chickpeas rinsed and drained
- 1/2 large yellow onion chopped
- 1/2 cup walnuts finely ground
- 1/2 cup old fashioned rolled oats
- 1/2 cup brown rice cooked
- 1 Tablespoon Nama Shoyu
- 2 teaspoons chili powder
- 2 Tablespoons ketchup
- 1/2 teaspoon salt
- 1 Tablespoon dried Italian seasoning

Sauce
- choose any mushroom or marinara sauce
- Squash or Zucchini Noodles
- goes perfect over a 1 cup of squash or zucchini noodles

Directions Meatballs
1. using a food processor pulse together chickpeas, onion, walnuts, rolled oats and brown rice until it looks like meal. Don't over pulse; there should be some chunks
2. spoon out the meatless meal and add to a container. Mix in chili powder, salt, pepper, Italian season and ketchup
3. if you prefer a smoother meatball, place meal back into the food processor and pulse more
4. using your hands make medium size balls, add each to a plate and set aside
5. coat the bottom of a baking sheet with oil
6. then place balls onto the baking sheet. Allow balls to bake for 15-20 minutes or until the balls are light brown

7. once done eat the balls as they are or add them to a sauce of choice and enjoy

9. FISH TACOS

Recipe by www.tastebetterfromscratch.com
Serves 4

Ingredients
- 1 pound lean white fish
- pinch salt
- 2 Tablespoons vegetable oil
- juice of 1 small lime
- 1 clove garlic minced
- 1 1/2 teaspoon chili powder
- 1 teaspoon ground cumin
- 1/2 teaspoon paprika
- Pinch Cayenne pepper

Shell
- 4 large Butter lettuce

Topping
- cashew sour cream
- 1-2 squeezes of a fresh lime
- fresh homemade salsa
- red onion
- avocado
- hot sauce *optional
- 2 Tablespoons red cabbage

Directions fish
1. season fish with a little salt and pepper on both sides
2. in a mixing bowl whisk together oil, lime juice, garlic, chili powder, cumin, paprika and cayenne

3. add fish to a large plastic bag and add marinade to the fish. Allow marinade to soak into fish for 30 minutes
4. remove the fish from the bag and sauté in a frying pan with a little oil
5. allow fish to sit for 15 minutes once done before creating taco

Directions for taco
1. pull lettuce leaves away from the center stalk in whole pieces, rinse well and pat them dry
2. spoon out sautéed fish and add toppings
3. when done, close the tack by folding in the edges of the lettuce
4. enjoy

10. VEGAN TACOS

Serves 4

Walnut meat Ingredients
- Follow directions under collard green burrito

Toppings Ingredients
- Fresh homemade salsa *follow directions under sauces and dressings
- Savory cashew cream *follow directions under sauces and dressings
- 2-3 Tablespoons Sliced avocado

Shell
- 4 large Romaine lettuce

Directions for burrito
1. cut the end of the lettuce off about 2 inches so that you have more of the soft leaf

2. vertically add walnut mixture down the center vein of the lettuce
3. top walnuts mixture, avocado, cashew and cream
4. when done, close the longest edges of the lettuce like a taco and Enjoy

11. BAKED SALMON PATTIES

Recipe by www.mommyshomecooking.com
Serves 6

Ingredients
- 6 Tablespoons water
- 2 Tablespoons golden flaxseed meal
- 18 ounce wild pink salmon about 3 cans
- 1/2 cup almond meal
- 1/2 cup fresh parsley chopped
- 1 shallot finely chopped
- 1 green onion sliced
- 1/2 teaspoon salt
- 1 teaspoon garlic powder
- 1/2 teaspoon dill
- 1/4 teaspoon black pepper
- 2 Tablespoons fresh lime juiced
- 2 Tablespoons olive oil

Directions
1. add flaxseed meal and water to a small bowl and stir. Then let it sit for 5 minutes so that it can thicken
2. remove salmon from the can. Pour off the water, rinse two to three times then remove from the can. Be sure to squeeze off excess water then add to a bowl
3. remove and discard excess skin and bones from the salmon so that you are left with only the salmon meat

4. crumble the salmon meat up and add the almond meal, parsley, shallot, green onion, salt, garlic powder, dill, black pepper, lime juice, flaxseed mixture and mix well
5. form 6 salmon patties
6. coat a baking sheet with olive oil and add each patty
7. bake patties for 15-20 minutes or until golden brown. Be sure to flip the patties to brown both sides
8. plate and enjoy

12. CAULIFLOWER RICE

Recipe by www.foodnetwork.com
Serves 4

Ingredients
- 1 large head cauliflower
- 3 Tablespoons olive oil
- 1 medium onion finely chopped
- pinch salt
- 2 Tablespoons fresh parsley finely chopped
- 1/2 fresh lemon juiced
- pinch

Directions
1. break cauliflower up into florets cutting away as much of the stem as possible
2. In a food processor pulse cauliflower until it resembles the size of couscous and set aside
3. add oil to a frying pan then spoon in onions and sauté until lightly brown
4. add cauliflower to the onions and mix in salt and pepper
5. stir frequently allowing cauliflower to soften
6. once done pour cauliflower into a bowl
7. squeeze on lemon juice and garnish with parsley
8. plate and enjoy

13. ROASTED CAULIFLOWER STEAK

Serves 4

Ingredients
- 1 Whole Cauliflower
- 1-2 Tablespoons Olive Oil
- pinch salt
- pinch black pepper
- 1 Tablespoon nutritional yeast
- 1/2 teaspoon fresh lime
- 2 cloves minced garlic

Directions
1. preheat oven to 400 degrees F
2. cut cauliflower in large 1/2-1 inch pieces. Rinse and pat dry
3. whisk together olive oil, salt, pepper, nutritional yeast, fresh lime and garlic
4. add cauliflower to a large plastic bag
5. pour marinade on top of cauliflower and allow it to sit for 30 minutes
6. coat a baking sheet with olive oil
7. add cauliflower steak to baking sheet so that it lays flat
8. poast for 10-15 minutes then brush cauliflower with a little more of the marinade
9. roast 10-15 minutes more until cauliflower is soft then remove from the oven
10. allow steak to cool then enjoy

14. VEGETARIAN CHILI

Recipe by www.cookieandkate.com
Serves 4-6

Ingredients
- 2 Tablespoons olive oil
- 1 medium onion
- 1 large red bell pepper
- 2 medium carrots chopped
- 2 ribs of celery chopped
- 1/2 teaspoon salt
- 4 cloves garlic minced
- 2 Tablespoons chili powder
- 2 teaspoons ground cumin
- 1 1/2 teaspoons smoked paprika
- 1 teaspoon dried oregano
- 2 15oz cans petite diced tomatoes
- 2 15oz can black beans
- 1 15oz can pinto beans
- 2 cups vegetable broth
- 1 dried bay leaf
- 2 Tablespoons fresh lime juiced
- garnish with cilantro

Directions
1. in a large pot warm olive oil and add vegetables onion, bell pepper, carrot and celery
2. sprinkle in 1/4 teaspoon salt and stir.
3. cook down until vegetable are soft about 10 minutes
4. then add garlic, chili powder, cumin, paprika and oregano; cook another minute
5. drain and rinse the black and pinto beans and add them to the pot along with tomatoes and their juices
6. allow to simmer for 5-10 minutes then add bay leaf and simmer another 10 minutes

7. to increase the thickness of the chili blend 1 cup in a blender then add back to pot
8. mix in cilantro, vinegar, salt, and pepper
9. allow chili to cool then enjoy

15. LENTIL BURGER

Serves 4-6

Ingredients
- 1/2 bag dried green lentils
- 1 whole yellow onion
- 4 cloves minced garlic
- onion powder
- garlic powder
- cumin
- 1/2 cup walnuts
- 1/2 cup rolled oats finely ground
- pinch salt
- pinch black pepper
- Italian seasoning

Directions Lentils
1. preheat oven to 400 degrees F
2. soak dried lentils in water for 24 hours then rinse and add to a pot with enough water to cover the top of the lentils by 3 inches
3. cook lentils for 1 - 2 hours until lentils are soft
4. once done allow them to drain in a colander and set them aside for later
5. boil sweet potato in water until it is soft. Peel off the skin and set it aside for later
6. using a food processor pulse walnuts and rolled oats until they are finely chopped

7. then add lentils, onion, garlic, sweet potato and rolled oats and pulse some more until they are mixed well
8. spoon out the lentils into a bowl and add additional spices including onion powder, garlic powder, black pepper and cumin
9. using your hands create small patties with your hands and set aside
10. coat a baking sheet with oil
11. add patties to baking sheet and bake for 15-20 minutes or until patties are light brown
12. once done set aside to cool for 10-15 minutes then Enjoy

16. VEGAN STEAK

Recipe by www.veggierose.com
Serves 4

Ingredients

Steak (Seitan)
- 1/2 cup vegetable stock
- 1/2 cup white beans
- 1 1/4 cup vital wheat gluten flour
- 2 Tablespoons tomato sauce
- 2 Tablespoons nutritional yeast
- 1 teaspoon paprika
- 1/2 teaspoon garlic powder
- 1/2 teaspoon onion powder
- 1/2 teaspoon black pepper
- 1/2 teaspoon sea salt

Marinade
- 6 teaspoons nama shoyu
- 1 teaspoon raw agave
- 1/2 teaspoon paprika

- 1/2 teaspoon onion powder
- 1/2 teaspoon garlic powder
- pinch black pepper

Broil Steak
- 4 Tablespoons olive oil
- 8-10 sprigs thyme
- 1 whole yellow thinly sliced onion
- pinch black Pepper
- 6 cloves garlic

Directions Steak
1. in a large mixing bowl add steak ingredients except for vegetable stock. Mix ingredients well
2. then add vegetable broth. If dough is stick add a bit more flour. If dough is dry add a bit more vegetable stock
3. once kneaded, divide the dough out into four equal parts. This will be your steak
4. take one of the parts and roll it out until it is a 1/4 inch steak. Do this for each dough part.
5. steam steak for 45 minutes

Direction for Marinade
1. combine all ingredients in a bowl then pour into a Ziploc bag
2. once the steaks are finished steaming, drain the water and add each one to the marinade
3. allow them to soak for 1 hour making sure to flip the bag every 15 minutes or so. This will ensure that the steak is evenly seasoned

Broil Steak
1. turn the oven to broil
2. coat the bottom of a baking sheet with oil

3. then add onion, garlic and thyme to baking sheet. Be sure to move the ingredients around while in the oven to keep them from burning
4. place steaks to the of onion, garlic and thyme and place in the broiler
5. allow steak to get golden brown on one side then flip
6. once done, remove steaks from broiler and top with onion, garlic and thyme
7. plate the steaks and enjoy

17. CAULIFLOWER MASH (RAW RECIPE)

Recipe by www.rawtarian.com
Serves 4

Ingredients
- 3 cups Cauliflower
- 1 Clove garlic
- 1/2 teaspoon Sea salt
- 1 cup Cashews
- 2 Tablespoons Water

Directions
1. add all ingredients to a food processor and pulse until smooth. You may be tempted to add more water but do not because your mash will be too watery. Instead scrape the sides of your food processor and pulse some more
2. spoon into a bowl and Enjoy

18. HAPPY HEALTHY RAW VEGAN NACHOS

Recipe by www.therawchef.com
Serves 4

Ingredients Spicy beans *add bullets

- 1 cup sunflower seeds soaked for 4 hours or more
- 1/2 cup sun-dried tomato soak water (reserved from soaking sun-dried tomatoes)
- 1 Tablespoon brown miso
- 2 teaspoons cumin
- 1teaspoon chipotle powder
- 2 teaspoon paparika
- 2 teaspoon ground coriander
- 1/4 cup water
- 1 teaspoon garlic powder
- 2 teaspoon onion powder
- 1 chili chopped & seeds removed
- 2 spring onions chopped
- 1/4 cup fresh coriander chopped

Ingredients Tomato sauce

- 1 cup sun-dried tomatoes soaked for at least 1 hour
- 1/2 cup sun-dried tomato soak water (reserved from soaking sun-dried tomatoes)
- 2 tomatoes chopped
- 1 Tablespoon lime juice
- 1 clove garlic
- 1/2 teaspoon salt

Directions Spicy beans

1. in a food processor, grind all ingredients except the last 2 until they bind together
2. then add the spring onions and coriander and pulse leaving some texture to the onion and coriander

3. sprinkle mixture directly onto a mesh dehydrator sheet leaving plenty of gaps between pieces of the mixture so the air can flow round nicely
4. dehydrate for 12 hours then place in a large bowl and set aside in preparation of the tomato sauce

Directions Tomato sauce
1. grind all ingredients in a food processor or blender until they form a thick but slightly chunky sauce
2. add to the bowl with the sunflower seed mixture then mix the two thoroughly

SALADS

1. SIMPLE CUCUMBER SALAD *DRESSING LEMON JUICE

Serves 1-2

Ingredients
- 2-3 medium cucumbers diced
- 1/4- 1/2 cup sweet cherry tomatoes
- 2 Tablespoon sliced black olives
- 2 Tablespoons olive oil
- pinch black pepper
- 1 teaspoon red onion
- 1-2 Tablespoons fresh lemon juiced

Directions
1. Petite dice cucumbers and add them to a bowl
2. Add all other ingredients and allow them to sit for 10 minutes
3. Then enjoy

2. FIESTA SALAD *DRESSING FRESH LIME JUICE

Serves 1-2

Ingredients
- 2-3 Tablespoons cup homemade guacamole*see recipe under sauces
- 2-3 Tablespoons diced homemade salsa* see recipe under sauces
- 2 Tablespoons Cilantro

- 1/4 cup black beans
- 2 Tablespoons yellow corn *optional
- 2 1/2 cups Romaine lettuce
- 1/2 cup arugula
- 1/2 fresh lime juice
- 1 pinch salt
- 1 pinch black pepper
- 2 Tablespoons pickled red onion
- 2 Tablespoons extra virgin olive oil

Directions

1. chop lettuce and arugula into bite size pieces and add to a bowl
2. spoon in guacamole, salsa, black beans and corn
3. then add pickled red onion, salt, pepper, olive oil and lime juice
4. mix well and enjoy

3. MEDITERRANEAN SALAD *DRESSING LEMON JUICE

Ingredients

- 1 large organic cucumbers diced
- 1/4 cup vine ripe tomatoes
- 4 Tablespoons can pitted black olives sliced
- 1/2 Fresh Lemon juiced
- 1/2 cup baby spinach
- 2 cups Romaine lettuce
- 1/4 cup chickpeas *from can or dried
- 2 teaspoons of apple cider vinegar
- 1 pinch salt
- 1 pinch black pepper
- 1 whole roasted red peppers
- 3-4 Tablespoons hummus
- 2 Tablespoons extra virgin olive oil

Directions

1. roast red bell pepper in the oven or use jarred roasted peppers
2. chop lettuce and spinach into bite size pieces and add to a bowl
3. then add cucumber, tomatoes, olives, chickpeas and red pepper
4. add the juice of a fresh lemon, olive oil, salt, and pepper
5. mix ingredients well
6. then spoon on humus and enjoy

4. HEAVENLY SOUL SALAD
*RICE WINE VINEGAR AND OLIVE OIL

Serves 3-4

Ingredients

- 2 cups black eyed peas if dried from bag or a 15 ounce can
- 1/2 medium red onion finely chopped
- 1 medium vine ripe tomato petite diced
- 1/2-1 whole red bell pepper finely chopped
- 1 teaspoon jalapeno pepper finely chopped
- 1/4 cup unseasoned rice wine vinegar
- 1 Tablespoon olive oil
- 1/4 teaspoon raw agave
- Pinch sea salt
- Pinch black pepper
- 1/4 dried parsley

Directions

Salad

1. place all ingredients into a bowl, mix well and Enjoy
2. garnish with parsley

Black eyed peas dried

1. pour out 1/2 bag of dried peas into a bowl
2. soak peas overnight
3. add peas to a pot with enough water to cover them by 3 inches
4. slow cook peas on medium heat until they are soft. This may take 2-3 hours. Add more water if needed
5. halfway through the cook add olive and a pinch of salt
6. once done, drain the water and add to a bowl in preparation for salad

5. VEGAN GREEK SALAD
*DRESSING LEMON JUICE AND OLIVE OIL

Serves 1-2

Ingredients

- 3 cups romaine lettuce chopped into medium size pieces
- 1/4 cup Kalamata pitted olives
- 1/2 vine ripe tomatoes petite diced
- 1/2 fresh lemon juiced
- 1 medium cucumber sliced thin
- pinch black pepper
- pinch Salt
- 1-2 Tablespoons olive oil

Tofu Feta Ingredients

- 1 package extra firm tofu diced into medium size cubes
- 1 Tablespoon nutritional yeast
- 1 Tablespoon oregano
- 1/2 cup apple cider vinegar
- 1/4 cup fresh lemon juiced

Directions

Tofu Feta

1. create a marinade by adding the fresh lemon juice, apple cider vinegar, oregano and nutritional yeast to a bowl
2. pour the marinade over the tofu and place in the refrigerator for two hours
3. remove a 1/2 cup of tofu feta for your Greek Salad

Salad

1. add all salad ingredients to a bowl and mix well
2. spoon on tofu feta
3. add spices to taste and Enjoy

6. SESAME NO FRY STIR-FRY

Serves 4

Ingredients

- 1/2 cup red cabbage finely chopped
- 1/2 cup green cabbage finely chopped
- 1 whole small zucchini quartered and sliced thin
- 1 large carrot grated
- 1/2 leek slice thin
- 3-4 cloves garlic minced or pressed
- 1/2 fresh lemon juiced
- 1-2 Tablespoons raw agave
- 1/2 teaspoon stone-ground mustard
- 1-2 teaspoons cold-pressed sesame oil
- 1 Tablespoon white sesame seeds
- 2 inch piece ginger minced or pressed
- 1/4 of a whole red and yellow bell pepper finely chopped
- 1/2 cup baby portabella mushroom sliced thin

Directions

1. add all ingredients to a bowl and mix well
2. allow bowl to sit for 10 minutes then Enjoy

7. AVOCADO, APPLE KALE SALAD *DRESSING LEMON VINAIGRETTE

Serves 2-3

Ingredients

- 2 cups chopped kale
- 1 cup chopped Romaine lettuce
- 2 ripe avocados diced
- 1 whole sweet red apple diced
- 1/4 cup baby tomatoes
- 1/8 teaspoon fresh lemon juiced
- 1 teaspoon sliced almonds

Directions

1. de-core, dice the red apple and add to a bowl. Then pour on fresh lemon juice and allow it to sit while other ingredients are being prepared
2. chop all other ingredients except almonds, add to bowl and mix well
3. spoon in apple, sprinkle on almonds and Enjoy

8. VEGAN CARROT TUNA SALAD

Serves 2-3

Equipment:
- Juicer. By using a juicer you are able to create the tuna like consistency

Ingredients
- 4-5 large organic carrots
- 1/2 medium white onion
- 1 whole organic celery stalk
- 2 Tablespoons of Veganaise
- 1 pinch of salt
- 1-2 Pinches of black pepper

Directions
1. rinse carrots over cool water
2. scrape each carrot until the outer layer of each is gone; each should be bright in color.
3. slice carrots so that they can easily be pushed through your juicer.
4. juice each carrot. Drink the juice at your leisure; the juice will not be used for this dish
5. remove the carrot pulp and place it into a bowl.
6. add your onion and celery to the carrot pulp.
7. add your remaining ingredients Veganaise, salt and pepper
8. mix well
9. add more ingredients from step 7 a little at a time until the desired consistency and taste is achieved.

SAUCES AND DRESSING

1. RAW VEGAN HOMEMADE SALSA

Recipe by www.thespruceeats.com
Serves 1-2

Ingredients
- 2 tomatoes
- 2 cloves minced garlic
- 1/4 sea salt
- 1 Tablespoon lime juice
- 2 Tablespoons fresh cilantro (cut into small pieces)
- 1 Tablespoon red onion
- 1/2 teaspoon cumin
- 1/2 teaspoon chili powder
- 1 teaspoon jalapeño pepper

Directions
1. petite dice tomatoes, onion, and jalapeño pepper and add them to a bowl
2. then add garlic and cilantro
3. add sea salt, cumin and chili powder
4. squeeze in fresh lime and mix well
5. allow ingredients to sit for 10 minutes then enjoy

2. RAW VEGAN GUACAMOLE

Recipe by www.lovingitvegan.com
Serves 3-4

Ingredients
- 3 ripe avocados
- 1/2 small red onion finely chopped

- 10 cherry tomatoes
- 1/4 cup cilantro
- 1/2 lime
- pinch Sea Salt
- pinch Black pepper

Directions

1. peel avocados, cut into pieces and add them to your food processor
2. then add onion and tomatoes
3. blend all ingredients until smooth
4. remove mixture from the food processor and spoon into a bowl
5. add remaining ingredients (cilantro, salt, pepper, lime) and mix well
6. allow ingredients to sit for 10 minutes then enjoy

3. CREAMY MUSHROOM SAUCE (RAW/VEGAN)

Recipe by www.natalienorman.com
Serves 1-2

Ingredients

- 2 Tablespoons raw tahini sauce
- 6 baby Portobello mushroom
- 1/2 cup fresh tomato
- 1 Tablespoon first cold press olive oil
- 2 Tablespoons juice of fresh lemon
- 1 teaspoon sea salt
- 2 Tablespoons dried basil leaves
- pinch black pepper
- pinch garlic powder
- pinch onion powder

Directions

1. gently rinse mushrooms, pat them dry and cut them up and add them to your high speed blender
2. add all remaining ingredients to your blender and blend until smooth
3. spoon out your sauce into a bowl, add more spices to meet your desired taste
4. allow sauce to sit for 10 minutes then enjoy *this sauce can be served warm, just heat in a sauce pan for a few minutes on low heat

4. RAW CASHEW SOUR CREAM

Recipe by www.simple-veganista.com
Serves 1-3

Ingredients

- 1 cup raw cashews
- 1/2 - 3/4 cup unsweetened almond milk
- juice of one whole fresh lemon
- 1 teaspoon apple cider vinegar
- pinch sea salt

Directions

1. add all ingredients to a high speed blender and blend until smooth
2. add sauce to a bowl; if needed using a teaspoon add water until desired consistency has been achieved *be careful not to overdo it
3. allow sauce to sit for 10 minutes then enjoy

5. RAW VEGAN CESAR DRESSING

Recipe by www.thevegan8.com
Serves 3-4

Ingredients
- 1/2 cup cashews
- 1/4 cup water
- 2 Tablespoons fresh lemon juice
- 1/2 teaspoon raw agave
- 3 Tablespoons nutritional yeast
- 2 large cloves of garlic
- 1/2 teaspoon dried parsley
- 1/2 teaspoon black pepper
- 1/2 teaspoon fine sea salt

Directions
1. add all ingredients to a high speed blender and blend until smooth
2. add dressing to a bowl. If needed using a teaspoon add water until desired consistency has been achieved *be careful not to overdo it
3. allow dressing to sit for 10 minutes then enjoy

6. CREAMY SESAME GINGER DRESSING

Recipe by www.veggieinspire.com
Serves 5-6

Ingredients
- 1/2 cup raw cashews
- 1/4 cup rice wine vinegar
- 1 teaspoon Nama Shoyu (raw soy sauce)
- 1 green onion finely chopped
- 2 teaspoons sesame oil

- 1 inch piece fresh ginger or 1/2 teaspoon of ground ginger
- 1 clove garlic
- 1-2 teaspoon 100% maple syrup
- pinch Sriarcha
- pinch sea salt
- pinch black pepper
- 1-2 Tablespoons of water

Directions
1. add all ingredients to a high speed blender and blend until smooth
2. add dressing to a bowl. If needed using a teaspoon add water until desired consistency has been achieved *be careful not to overdo it
3. allow dressing to sit for 10 minutes then enjoy

7. RAW LEMON VINAIGRETTE

Recipe from www.thespruceeats.com
Serves 2-4

Ingredients
- 1 clove garlic
- 1 teaspoon Dijon mustard
- 2 Tablespoons first cold press olive oil
- 1/4 cup fresh lemon juiced
- 1/2 Tablespoon dried basil
- 2 Tablespoons fresh parsley finely chopped
- pinch sea salt
- pinch pepper

Directions

1. add all ingredients to a high speed blender and blend until smooth
2. add dressing to a bowl. If needed using a teaspoon add water until desired consistency has been achieved *be careful not to overdo it
3. allow dressing to sit for 10 minutes then enjoy

8. RAW VEGAN TOMATO MARINARA

Recipe by www.veggiesdontbite.com
Serves 2-3

Ingredients

- 1 cup sun dried tomatoes
- 4 medium sweet vine ripe tomatoes
- 2 cups cherry tomatoes
- 2 Tablespoons fresh thyme
- 2 green onions
- pinch Himalayan pink salt
- pinch lemon pepper
- pinch garlic powder

Directions

1. add all ingredients to a high speed blender and blend until smooth
2. add sauce to a bowl. If needed using a teaspoon add water until desired consistency has been achieved *be careful not to overdo it
3. allow sauce to sit for 10 minutes then enjoy

9. SAGE AND PEPPER MUSHROOM GRAVY

Recipe by www.thespruceeats.com
Serves 2

Ingredients
- 2 cups Shitake mushrooms
- 1/4 cup yellow onion
- 1/2 cup water
- 2 Tablespoons first cold press olive oil
- 2 teaspoons Nama Shoyu (raw soy sauce)
- 1 teaspoon nutritional yeast
- 1 teaspoon rubbed sage
- 1/2 teaspoon dried thyme
- pinch celery seed
- pinch black pepper

Directions
1. add all ingredients to a high speed blender and blend until smooth
2. add gravy to a bowl. If needed using a teaspoon add water until desired consistency has been achieved *be careful not to overdo it
3. allow gravy to sit for 10 minutes then enjoy

10. MAC & CHEESE SAUCE

Recipe by www.livesimplynatural.com
Serves 4

Ingredients
- 1 cup raw cashews
- 1 cup water
- 3 sun dried tomatoes
- 1/2 cup nutritional yeast

- 1 Tablespoon first cold press olive oil
- 1 teaspoon pink Himalayan salt
- 1 clove garlic
- 1/2 teaspoon onion powder
- 1/4 teaspoon turmeric

Directions

1. add all ingredients to a high speed blender and blend until smooth
2. add sauce to a bowl. If needed using a teaspoon add water until desired consistency has been achieved *be careful not to overdo it
3. allow sauce to sit for 10 minutes then enjoy

11. CASHEW CREAM

Recipe by www.thefullhelping.com
Serves 1-3

Basic

- 1 cup cashews
- 1/2 - 3/4 cup of water depending on desired consistency
- 1/4 teaspoon salt

Directions

1. add all ingredients to a high speed blender and blend until smooth
2. add ingredients to a bowl. If needed using a teaspoon add water until desired consistency has been achieved *be careful not to overdo it
3. allow ingredients to sit for 10 minutes then enjoy

Sweet

- 1 teaspoon vanilla extract
- 1-2 teaspoon maple syrup

- 1/4 teaspoon cinnamon
- 1inch piece ginger
- 1/4 teaspoon cardamom

Directions

1. add additional ingredients and follow directions under "basic" section

Savory

- 2 teaspoons fresh lemon juiced
- 1 clove garlic
- pinch paprika
- pinch onion powder

Directions

1. add additional ingredients and follow directions under "basic" section

SNACKS: SALTY/SAVORY

1. SPICY OKRA POPCORN

Serves 1-2

Eat this Raw to enjoy the greatest amount of nutrients or crispy

Ingredients
- 1 cup raw okra sliced thin
- pinch sea salt
- pinch cayenne pepper
- pinch garlic powder
- pinch onion powder
- pinch smoked paprika
- 1/2 teaspoon nutritional yeast

Directions
1. slice okra into thin pieces and add them to a bowl
2. sprinkle on spices
3. mix ingredients well and enjoy

Crispy Okra Popcorn
4. preheat oven to 450 degrees F
5. using olive oil coat the bottom a baking sheet
6. slice okra into thin pieces and add them to a bowl
7. sprinkle on spices
8. mix ingredients well and add them to baking sheet
9. move pieces around using a spoon to avoid burning the okra
10. cook for 10 minutes or until desire crispiness is achieved

2. HUMMUS AND RAW VEGGIES

Serves 2-3

Ingredients Hummus
- 1/2 bag of dried chickpeas or 15oz can thoroughly rinsed chickpeas
- 1/4 cup fresh lemon juiced
- 1/4 cup raw tahini
- 1 small clove garlic
- pinch paprika
- pinch salt
- pinch black pepper
- 1/4 teaspoon cumin
- 1/4 -1/2 cup water

Directions using dried chickpeas
1. soak chickpeas for 24 hours
2. add to a saucepan on medium heat with enough water to cover them by 3 inches
3. slow cook chickpeas until they are soft; this may take 2-3 hours
4. once halfway cooked add olive oil to water as well as a pinch of salt and complete cooking
5. when done remove chickpeas and follow hummus recipe

Directions Hummus
1. add chickpeas to a food processor and other ingredients to a food processor except for paprika
2. then add water
3. process until smooth
4. spoon hummus out into a bowl
5. add more spices if desired
6. add paprika last with a drizzle of olive oil
7. allow hummus to sit for 10 minutes then Enjoy
8. eat hummus with your favorite vegetables

3. BAKED ZUCCHINI CHIPS

Recipe by www.aspicyperspective.com
Serves 3-4

Ingredients
- 4 Large Zucchini chips sliced to 1/8 of an inch
- 2 Tablespoons olive oil
- 1/2 teaspoon smoked paprika *optional
- 1/2 teaspoon cumin*optional
- Pinch salt

Directions
1. preheat oven to 230 degrees F
2. coat the bottom of a baking sheet with a thin layer of olive oil
3. add zucchini to the baking sheet
4. sprinkle on spices
5. cook for 1-2 hours or until desired crispiness has been achieve
6. remove from oven zucchini from oven, allow to cool and enjoy

4. ALMOND CRACKERS

Recipe by www.elanapantry.com
Serves 3-4

Ingredients
- 1 cup almond flour
- 3 Tablespoons water
- 2 Tablespoon golden flax meal
- 1 Tablespoon olive oil
- 1 Tablespoon finely chopped thyme
- 1/2 teaspoon fine sea salt

Directions
1. combine all ingredients in a large bowl
2. press dough between two pieces of parchment paper and roll out until it is 1/4 inch thick
3. Remove top of parchment paper and place the bottom portion of the dough on a baking sheet
4. Cut into 2 inch squares with a knife or pizza cutter
5. Bake at the lowest temperature possible on your oven until crunchy
6. once done, allow it to cool and enjoy

SNACKS: SWEET RAW VEGAN

1. CHOCOLATE BROWNIES

Recipe by www.minimalistbaker.com
Yields 12 brownies

Ingredients Brownies
- 1 1/2 cups raw walnuts
- 1 cup of raw almonds
- 2 1/4 cups pitted dates soaked
- 3/4 cups cacao powder
- 1/4 teaspoon sea salt
- 2 Tablespoons of cacao nibs

Ingredients Frosting
- 1/4 cup unsweetened almond milk
- 1 cup dairy-free dark chocolate
- 2 Tablespoons coconut oil
- 1/4 teaspoon sea salt

Directions Brownies
1. soak dates in water for 30 minutes with enough water to cover the top of them and set aside
2. add to food process and process until it is in small bits then place in a separate bowl for later use
3. clean out the food processor and add nuts; finely grind walnuts and almonds
4. then add cacao powder and sea salt and pulse to combine
5. then add dates a little at a time until ingredients are thick and doughy
6. remove chocolate dough to square container
7. knead in cacao nibs

8. flatten dough out until it is 1/4 - 1/2 inch thick
9. place in the freezer for 5-10 minutes then remove

Directions Frosting
1. add chocolate to a bowl and set aside
2. add almond milk to a sauce pan and heat until simmering
3. pour almond milk onto chocolate and mix until smooth
4. allow to sit for 2 minutes at room temperature
5. using a wood or rubber spoon stir in salt, coconut oil. Mix until smooth
6. set in the freezer for 10 minutes or until the chocolate thickens
7. generously cover the whole brownie with frosting and sprinkle with left over walnuts
8. place back in the freezer for 5 minutes then remove and Enjoy

2. WALNUT-OATMEAL DOUGH BITES

Recipe inspired by www.runningonrealfood.com
Yields 25 bites

Ingredients
- 3/4 cups pitted dates soaked
- 2 cups old fashioned rolled oats
- 1 teaspoon cinnamon
- 2/3 cups almond butter
- 1/4 cup 100% maple syrup
- 1 teaspoon vanilla extract
- 1/2 teaspoon sea salt
- 1/4 cup finely chopped walnuts

Directions
1. add walnuts to a food processor and finely chop
2. place onto parchment paper and set to the side

3. rinse processor and add all other ingredients to the food processor
4. process until smooth and doughy. Dough may feel warm to the touch
5. using your hands create medium size dough balls
6. place each ball one at a time on parchment paper with walnuts
7. light coat each ball and place into a separate container
8. once all done, place balls in the freezer for 5 minutes
9. remove and enjoy

3. HOMEMADE APPLESAUCE

Recipe by www.draxe.com
Serves 3-4

Ingredients
- 3 Apple peeled, cored and sliced
- 1 teaspoon Fresh lemon juice
- 1 teaspoon cinnamon

Directions
1. place all ingredients into a blender
2. blend for 2-3 minutes. You may need to spoon water a little at a time until desired consistency is achieved
3. remove, chill if desired and enjoy

4. MINI APPLE PIE BITES

Recipe by www.eatingbirdfood.com
Yields 10-15 bites

Apple Filling
- 3 medium red apples
- 3/4 cup pitted dates soaked
- 1/2 teaspoon cinnamon
- 1/2 teaspoon sea salt
- pinch ground nutmeg
- 1/2 teaspoon fresh lemon squeezed
- 3/4 - 1 cup water

Crust
- 1 cup pitted dates
- 1/2 cup unsweetened shredded coconut
- 1/2 cup raw almonds

Directions apple filling
1. soak dates in enough water to cover them for 30 minutes
2. remove the skin, de-core and petite dice apples
3. pour fresh lemon over apples and set aside
4. once dates are done pour off water and add them to a food processor
5. then add spices cinnamon, salt nutmeg and fresh water a little at time until dates are able; process smoothly (start with 1/2 cup). liquid should be pourable syrup
6. add more water if needed
7. once done pour syrup onto apples and allow it to sit while preparing the crust

Directions Crust
1. soak dates with enough water to cover them for 30 minutes

2. once done, add dates, coconut and almonds to a food processor
3. process until crust is stick
4. place plastic wrap over a mini cupcake pan; push plastic down so that crust can sit in each one.
5. Using your hands add sticky crust one by one to your cupcake holder. Push down and
6. shape it to fit mini cupcake space
7. once done place in the freeze for 15 minutes to allow ingredients to come together
8. remove the crust and spoon on the filling
9. place back into the freezer for another 15 minutes
10. remove and enjoy

5. RAW VEGAN CHOCOLATE MOUSSE

Recipe by www.tastykitchen.com
Serves 3

Ingredients
- 1 cup raw cashews *soaked for 24 hours
- 2 Tablespoons raw agave
- 4 teaspoons coconut oil
- 1 whole vanilla bean
- 1/2 cup water
- 2 Tablespoons raw cacao powder

Directions
1. place all ingredients into food processor
2. process until smooth. you may need to spoon in water a little at a time until desired consistency is achieved
3. remove, chill if desired and enjoy

ABOUT THE AUTHOR

M etra is the founder and CEO of the premier fitness and yoga studios, Kinetics Personal Training & Group Fitness™, Kinetics Flow Hot Yoga & Aerial Fitness™, and Moving Meetings™ – their mobile sister company. Through the development of a team of certified personal trainers, yoga, aerial and group fitness instructors, Metra has led the growth of Kinetics and helped thousands of clients achieve personal transformation. Metra uses "whole-concept thinking" to transform, educate and motivate clients to reach their greatest potential.

Trailblazer in her own right, Metra has facilitated the growth of others using her signature coaching program designed to liberate and empower others to push past limiting beliefs and gain access to the best versions of themselves. For over a decade, Metra has successfully developed a "train to lead" culture – a way of being that encourages her clients and staff to elevate others while individual personal achievements are being made.

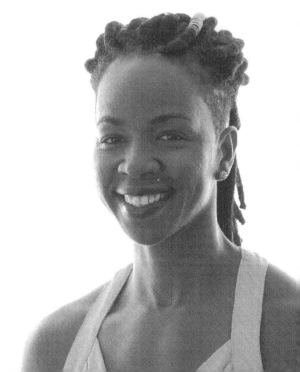

\

Made in the USA
Lexington, KY
09 December 2019